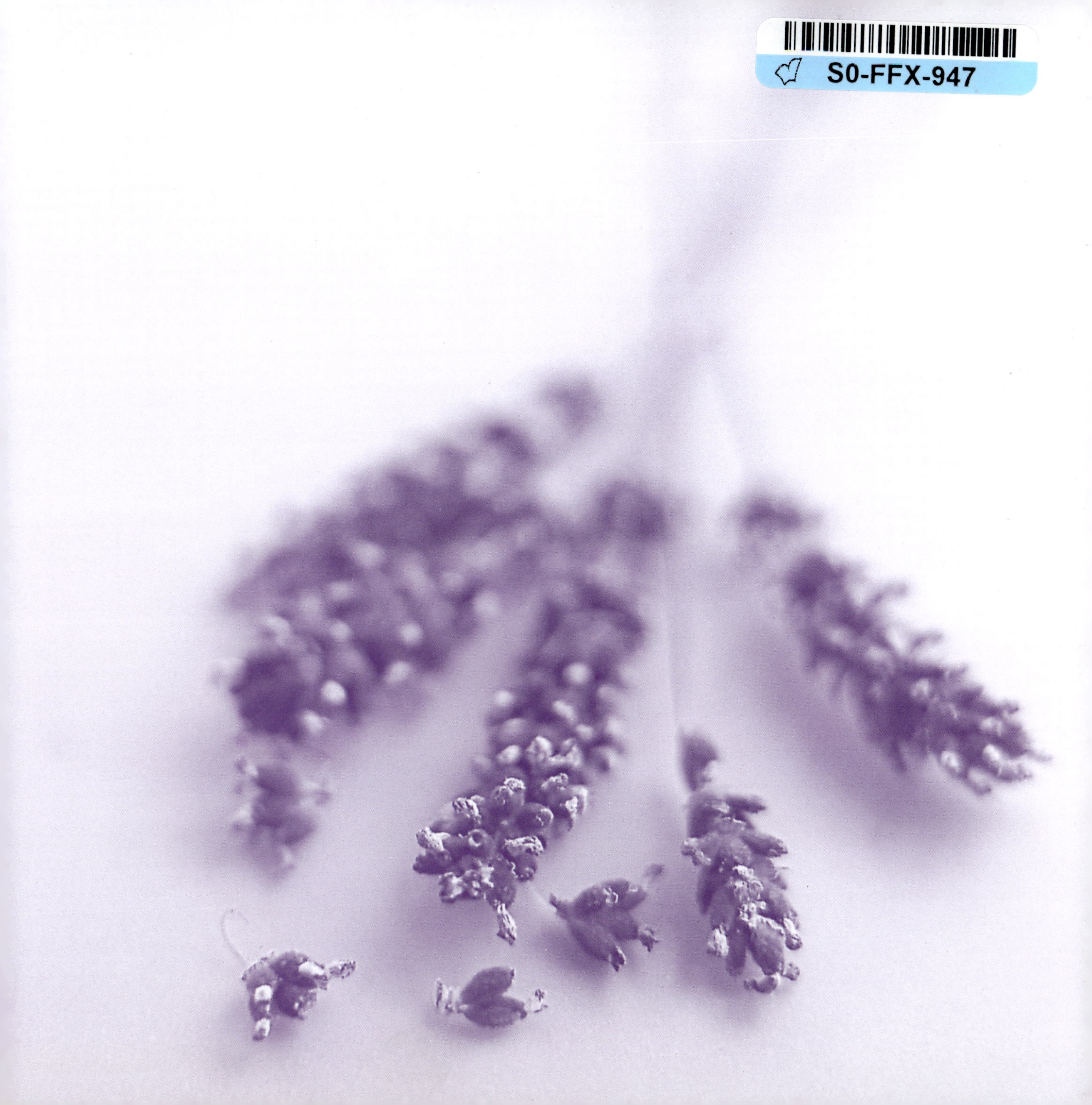

scent therapy

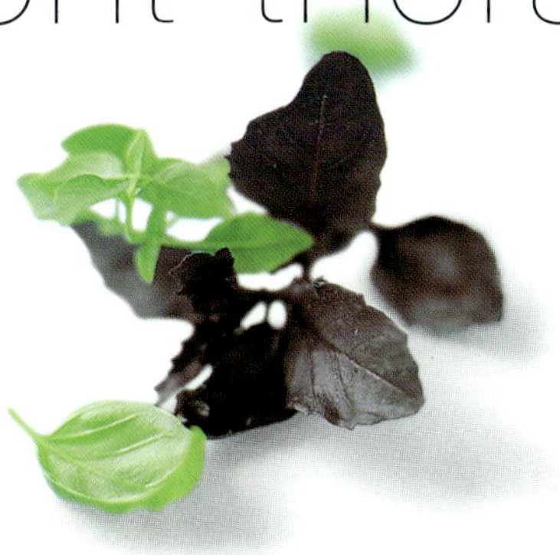

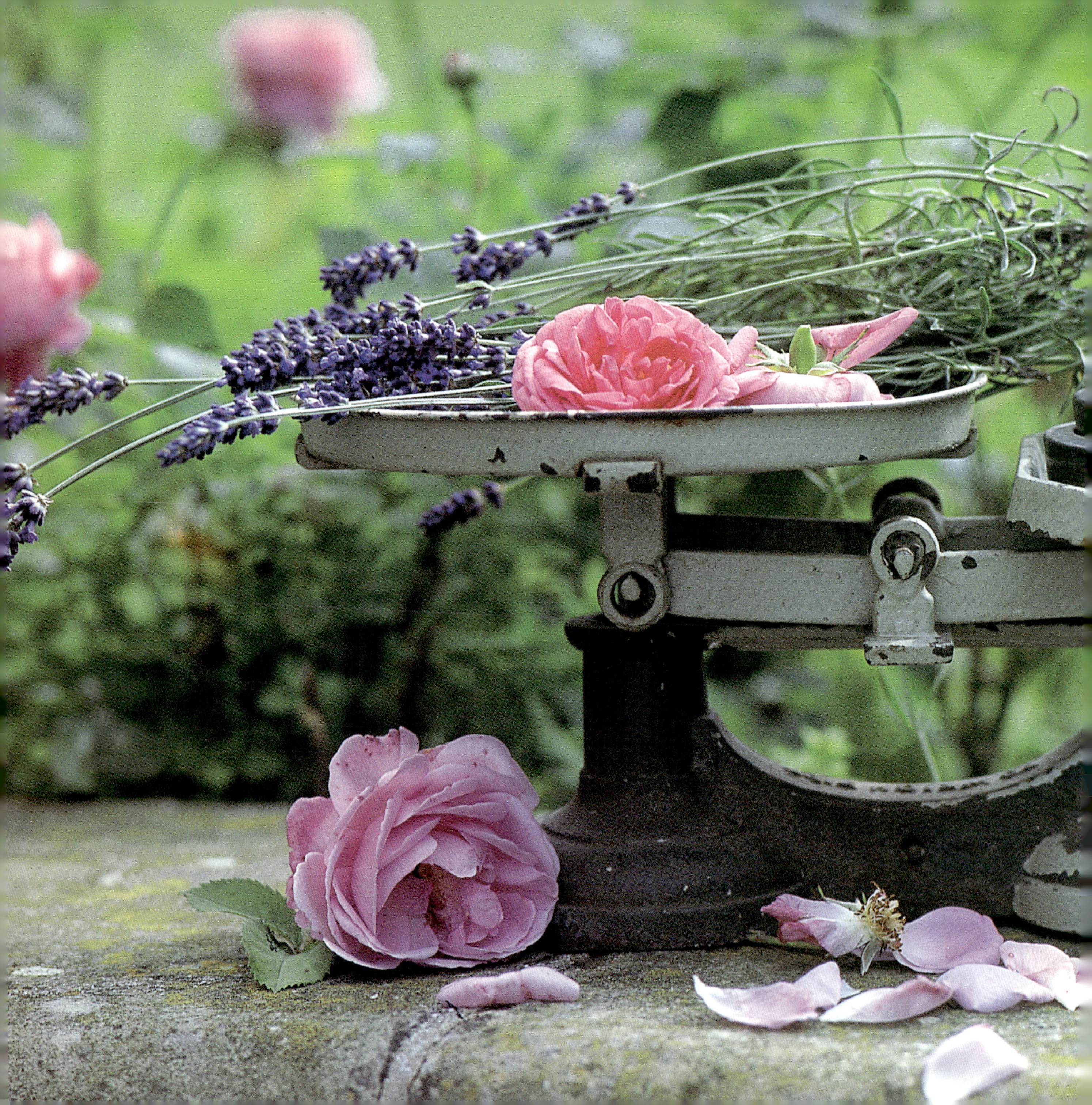

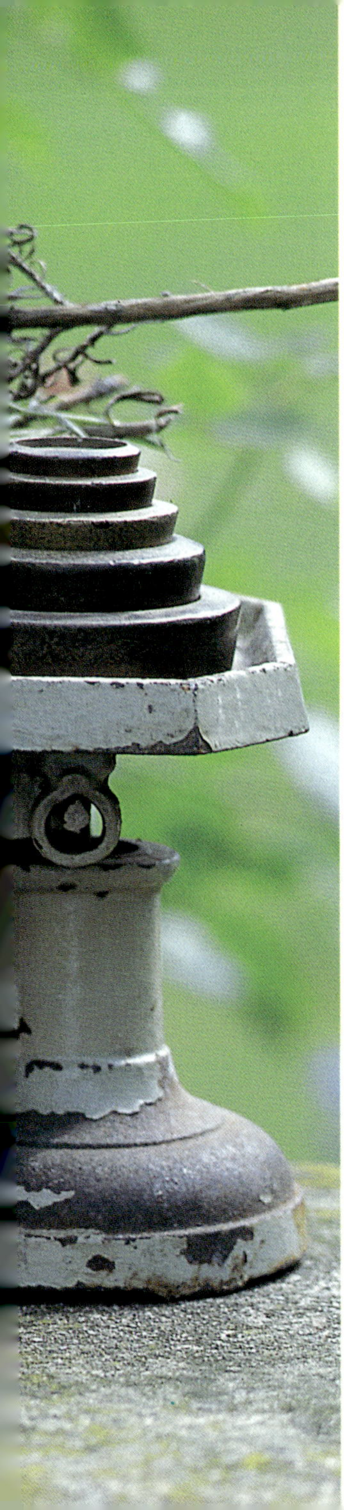

scent therapy

health and wellbeing through fragrance

Raje Airey

LORENZ BOOKS

First published by Lorenz Books in 2001

Lorenz Books is an imprint of
Anness Publishing Limited
Hermes House
88–89 Blackfriars Road
London SE1 8HA

Published in the USA by Lorenz Books
Anness Publishing Inc.
27 West 20th Street, New York, NY 10011

www.lorenzbooks.com

This edition distributed in Canada by Raincoast Books,
9050 Shaughnessy Street, Vancouver, British Columbia V6P 6E5

A CIP catalogue record for this book is available from the British Library

Publisher: Joanna Lorenz
Managing Editor: Linda Fraser
Senior Editor: Margaret Malone
Designer: Mark Latter
Proof Reader: Hayley Kerr
Production Controller: Yolande Denny

10 9 8 7 6 5 4 3 2 1

Publisher's note: The reader should not regard the ideas, recommendations and techniques expressed and described in this book as substitutes for the advice of a qualified medical practitioner. Any use to which the recommendations, ideas and techniques are put is at the reader's sole discretion and risk.

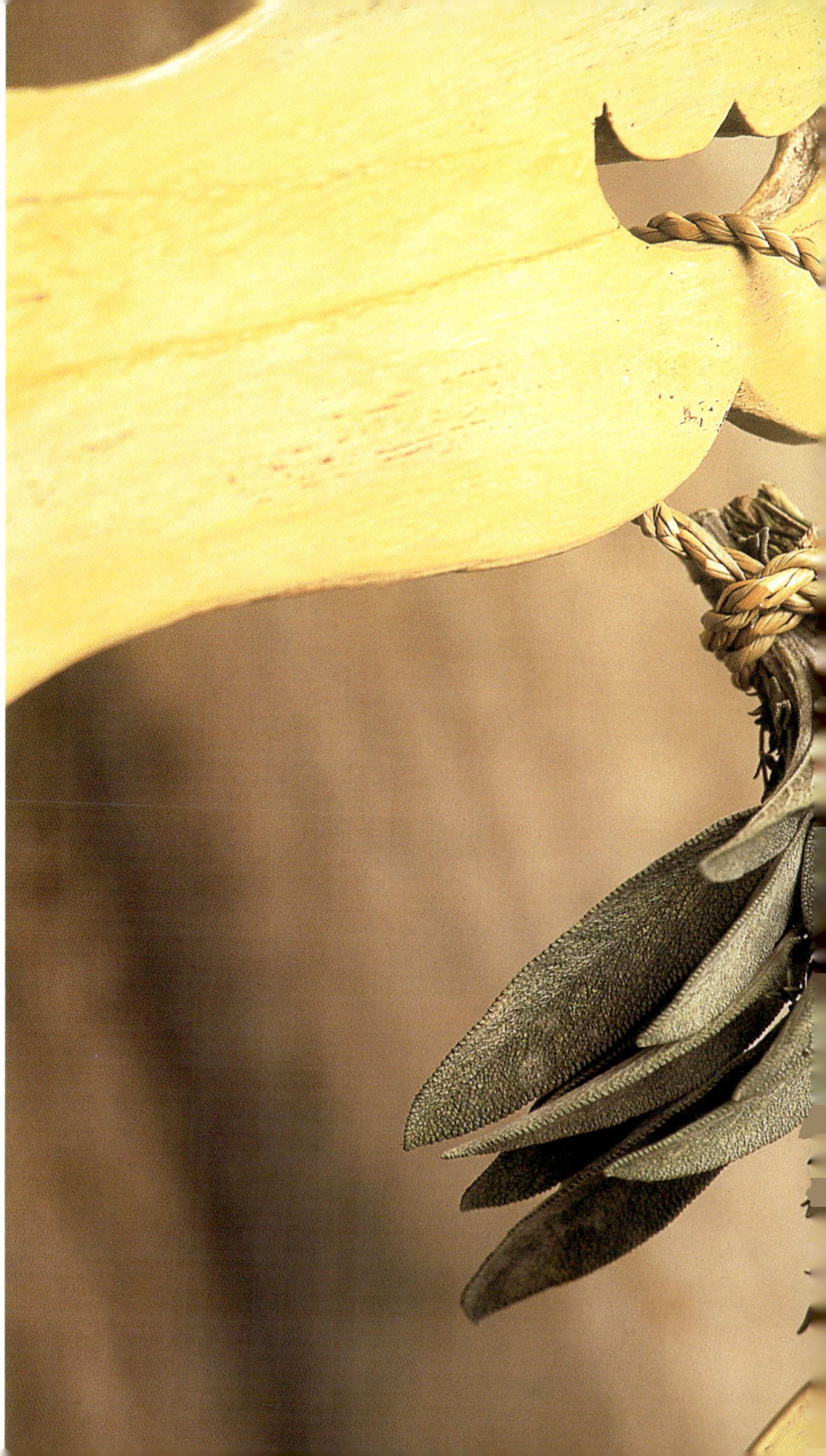

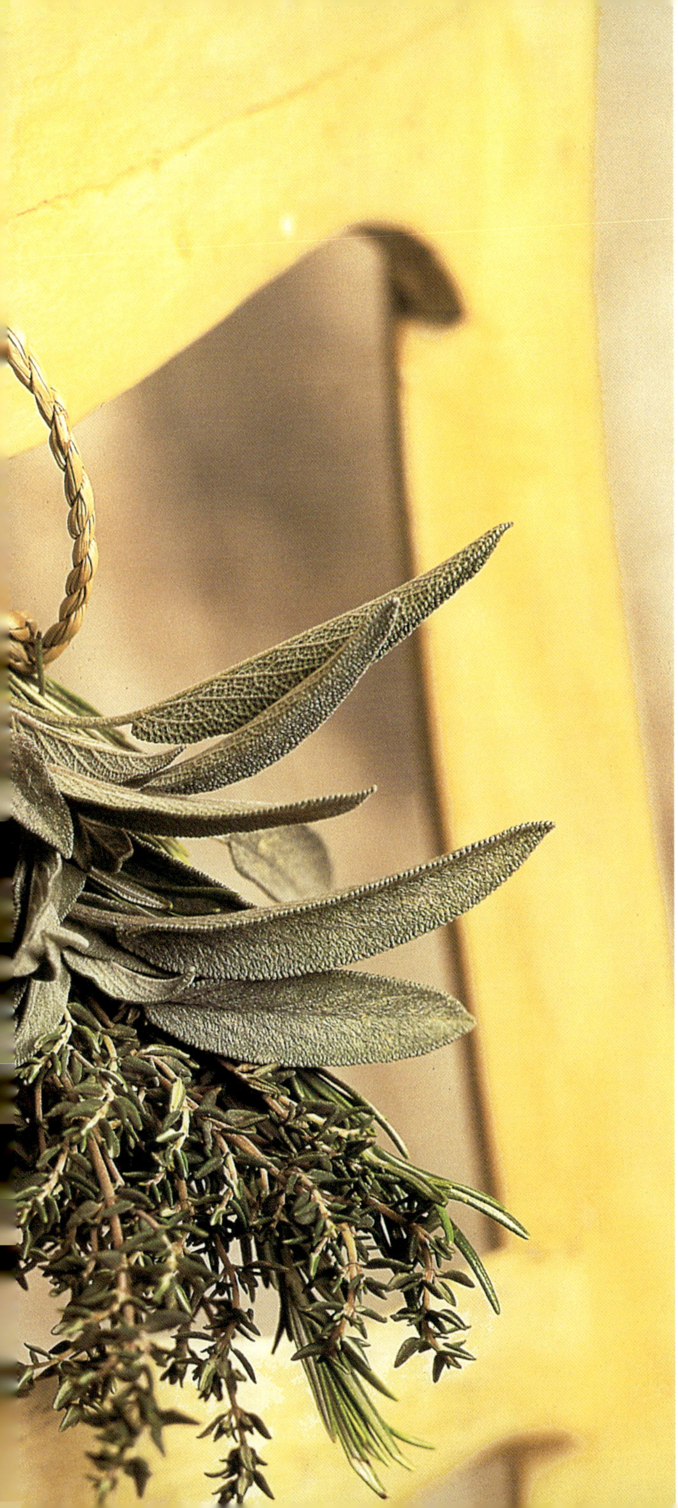

contents

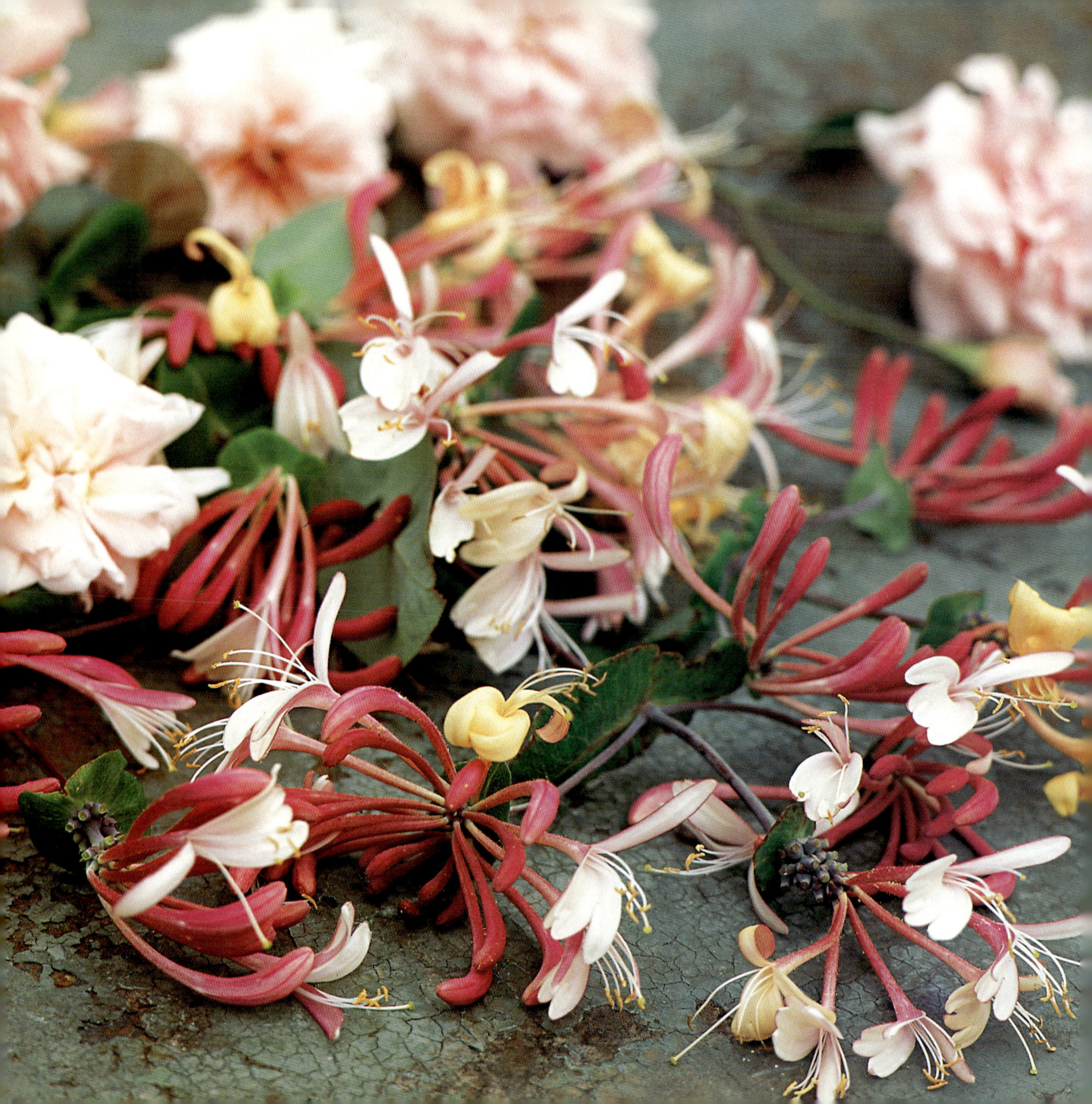

introduction

Every day we benefit from sweet aromas, often in subtle ways that go unnoticed. Yet the ability of scent to affect our moods and enhance aspects of our lives is well recorded. Throughout history, people have utilized scents for their healing, cleansing and preservative properties, as well as appreciating the sheer pleasure they bring. Today, these properties are being rediscovered as we reconsider our approach to health and wellbeing, and search for an antidote to the pressures of modern life. Be it a bouquet of fresh flowers, the use of fresh herbs in cooking, or a massage with essential oils, these potent aromas are nature's gift to mind, body and spirit.

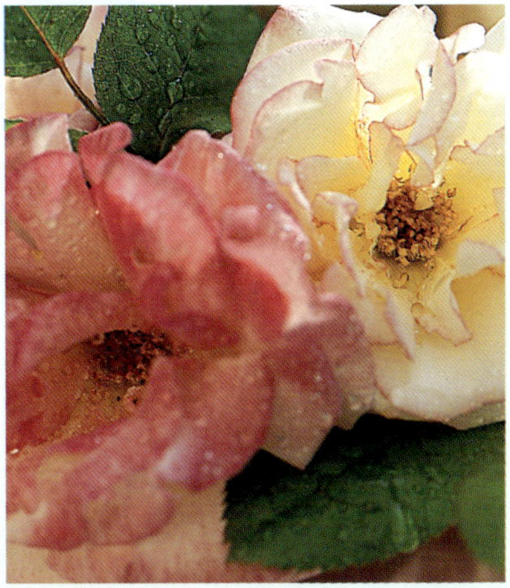

the power of scent

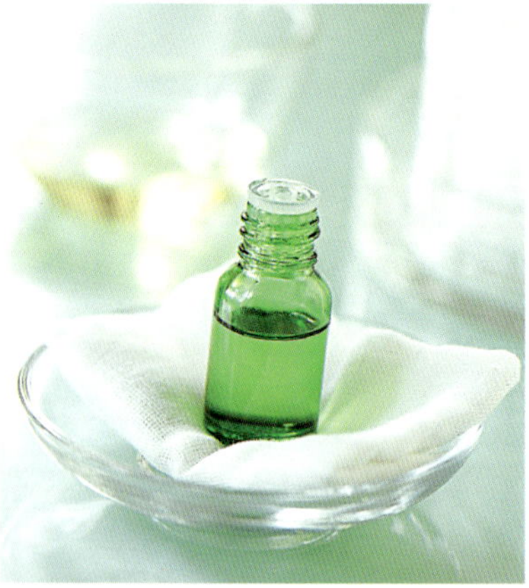

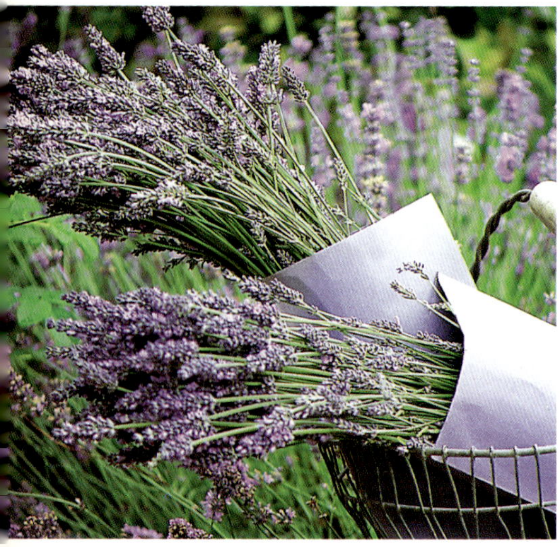

above and opposite The fragrance and character of a plant's essential oil is as individual and unique as the person using it.
top Aromatherapy seeks to harness the healing properties of essential oils contained within plants.

We all recognize how certain scents have the ability to evoke memories or arouse an instant emotional reaction, and there are countless episodes throughout history where the power of fragrance has been harnessed for a specific end: Cleopatra's lavish use of aromatics is credited with the seduction of both Julius Caesar and Mark Antony; and Louis XIV impressed guests at dinner parties by releasing doves drenched in perfume to scent the air around them.

Our sense of smell is registered in one of the oldest parts of the brain, known as the limbic area. This area is connected with memory, emotion and instinctive activities, such as sexual response, sleep, hunger and thirst. When we breathe in a scent, the aromatic molecules are quickly inhaled via the millions of sensitive cells that line the nasal passages, triggering messages that pass directly to the brain. This action causes chemical changes in the body, which affect many of the body's vital parts, from tissues and organs to body fluids and cells, as well as affecting the emotional state and spiritual aspects of the person. Consequently, scents can be used to positively influence our wellbeing – through direct application to the body or inhalation, by scenting the air around us, or by using in food and drinks.

The majority of these therapeutic scents originate in the plant world, which houses an abundance of aromas. They are produced by the aromatic oils contained in all parts of a plant, including the wood, bark, root, buds, seeds, leaves, fruit and flowers. The oils have an important role in the plant's survival as a species, and are described as the life-blood of the plant because of their "essential" nature. Each of these oils has a unique fragrance and character, and understanding how these characteristics work, and using them to our advantage, is the aim of scent therapy.

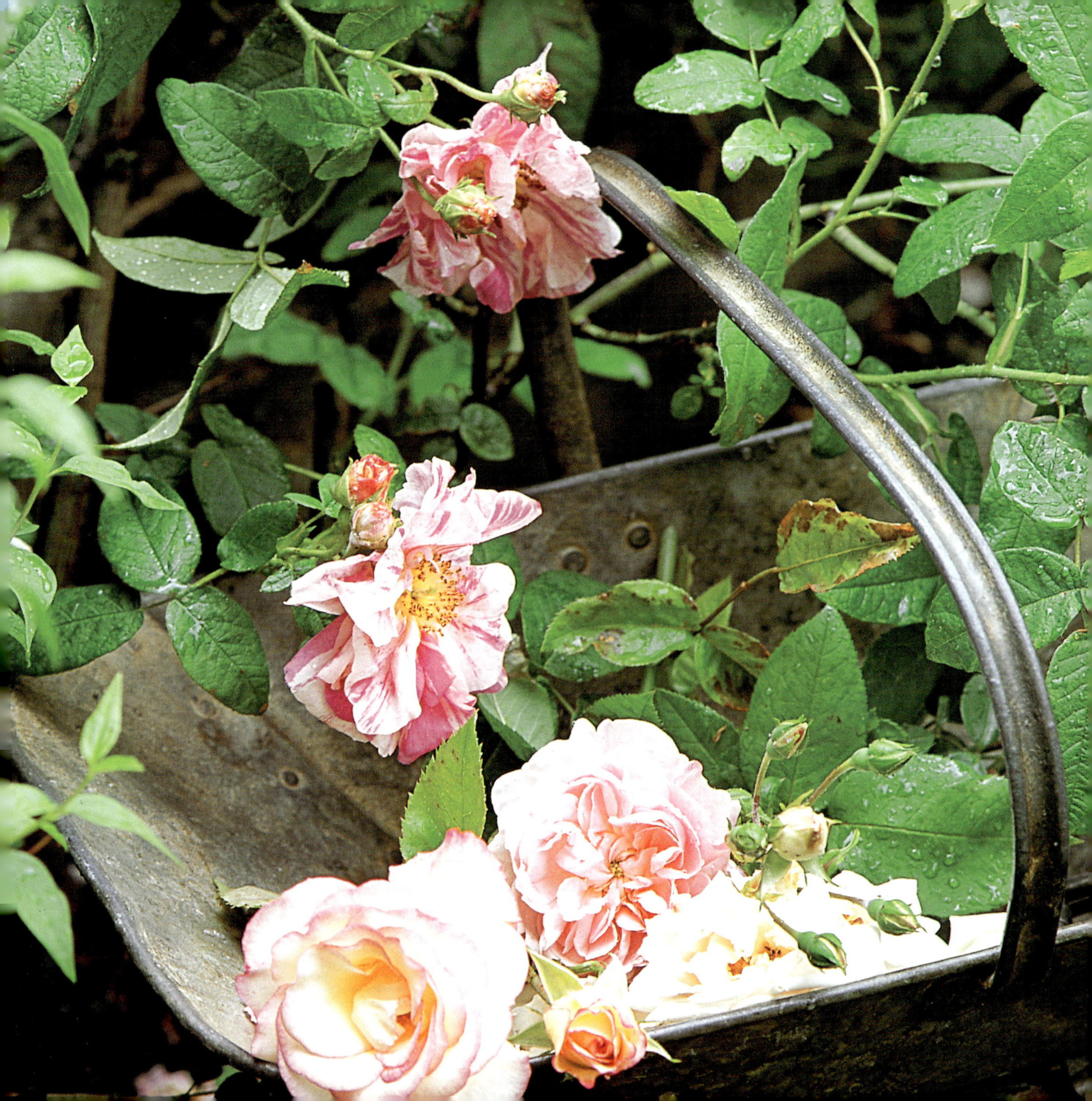

an ancient art

Scented products have been used by men and women since time began. More than 100,000 years ago, the Neanderthals made offerings of pollen and flowers to their dead, while around 7000 BC, people combined olive and sesame oils with plant fragrance to produce ointments. The use of plant oils is recorded in some of the earliest Chinese writings, in the Vedic manuscripts from India around 2000 BC, in Egyptian papyri from 1500 BC and in both the Old and New Testament stories in the Bible.

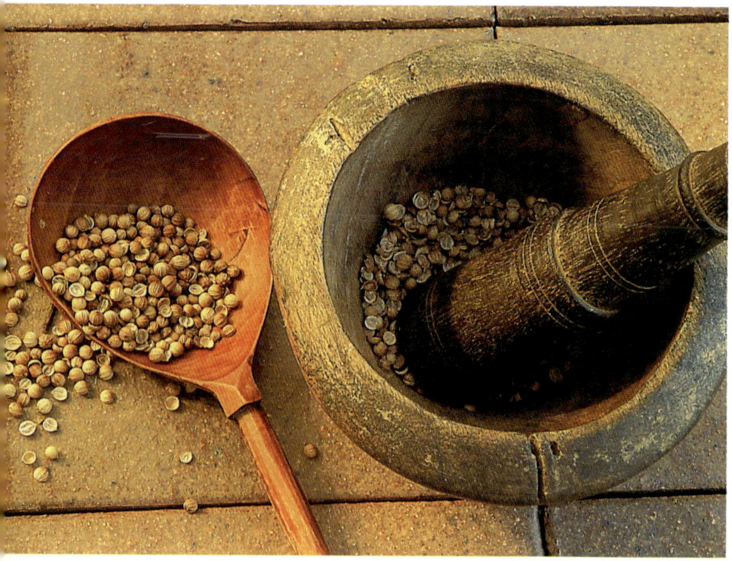

above Coriander has been valued as a flavouring and medicine since ancient times: among the riches found in the tombs of Pharaohs were coriander seeds. **opposite** Traditionally, herbs from the kitchen garden such as parsley, sage, rosemary and thyme are collected and tied into bundles and then hung up indoors to dry out. The dried leaves are used in cooking.

Early societies throughout the world recognized that aromas were powerful substances, possessing seemingly magical properties. In fact, the word "perfume" derives from the Latin *per fume*, meaning "through smoke", referring to the burning of aromatic herbs and resinous woods in ritual and healing. In Japan, *kodo* (perfumery) was a sacred art and special schools were set up to teach it. Ceremonial ways of burning incense were taught, as well as complex story dances for incense-burning rituals. In the Native American tradition, bundles of fragrant herbs such as sage were burned for protection and to clean energy fields or auras. This ritual, which is known as "smudging", is still carried out today.

The early use of scents for therapeutic and medicinal purposes was also widespread. The ancient Egyptians, Greeks and Romans built up extensive knowledge of the healing properties of plants and were skilled in the ways of preparing and using healing oils and unguents. In medieval Europe, the apothecary prepared and traded medicines made from exotic spices, resins and aromatics, imported from the East, and from the humble plants of the local countryside. There was a universal belief in the great power of fragrance to protect from disease, which led to the production of pomanders, the use of posies, strewing herbs and herbal fumigation. During the Great Plague, cedar, cypress, pine, sage, rosemary and thyme were burned in an attempt to keep the epidemic at bay.

However, although scents were considered precious commodities, with ceremonial significance and healing properties, they were also associated with beauty, sensuality and pampering. Wealthy women in ancient Egypt, for example, wore perfumed wax cones in their hair, which would slowly melt and cover the head and shoulders with perfume (and wax!), while at the height of the Roman civilization, there were more than one thousand bath houses in Rome, each offering massages with richly-scented oils. The Emperor Nero himself is said to have bathed in pure rose water, a favour he would sometimes bestow on guests.

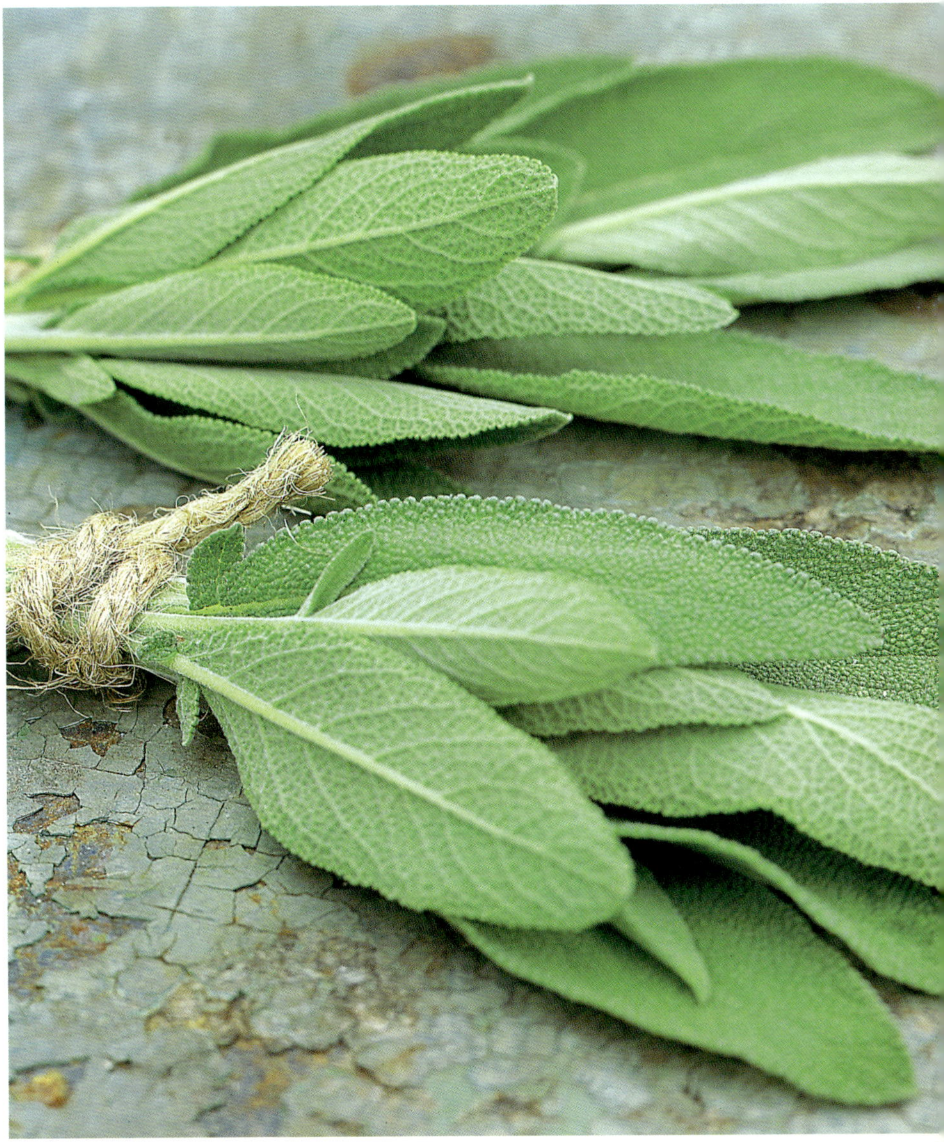

a modern appreciation

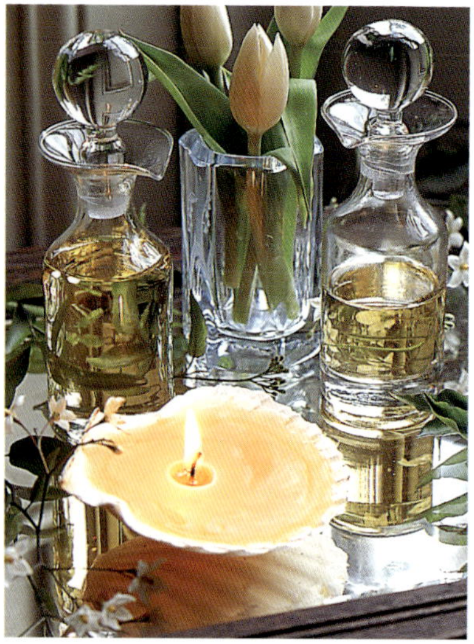

above In the 19th century, the use of scented lotions and oils increased as the knowledge and commercialization of perfumery developed.
opposite Lavender has traditionally been linked with the laundering of linens, and a pile of softly scented linens is just as pleasurable as it ever was.

After the fall of the Roman Empire in the 5th century the use of essential oils died out for a time in Europe. Elsewhere, however, the art flourished. In the 11th century, Arabia became the world centre for the production of perfume when Avicenna, a learned scientist, became the first to successfully distil rose essence since ancient times. This rich, heady perfume, known as attar of roses, was brought back to Europe by the Crusaders, and with it the secrets of perfumery.

The Renaissance gave further impetus to the detailed analysis and study of essential oils and other aromatic substances but, as scientific knowledge grew, the natural holistic philosophy of earlier ages was left behind. The use of synthetic and chemical drugs soon predominated over the use of herbs and oils in medicine, and scented products were considered of interest to perfume manufacturers only.

It wasn't until the early 20th century that a significant revival of interest in the healing properties of plants developed; much of it due to the curiosity shown by perfumers. René-Maurice Gattefossé, a French chemist, first coined the term *aromathérapie* in 1937 as a result of his investigations into the therapeutic properties of essential oils. Another Frenchman, Jean Valnet, also a doctor and scientist, used essential oils to treat wounds during World War II, and afterwards to treat specific illnesses. Elsewhere, others were rediscovering the benefits of using essential oils in massage, as practised by the ancient healers.

Since then, our knowledge of scents, and how to use them to address mental, physical and spiritual needs, has grown considerably. Accompanying these changes in attitude and developments in research has been a renewed appreciation for the knowledge left us by ancient societies.

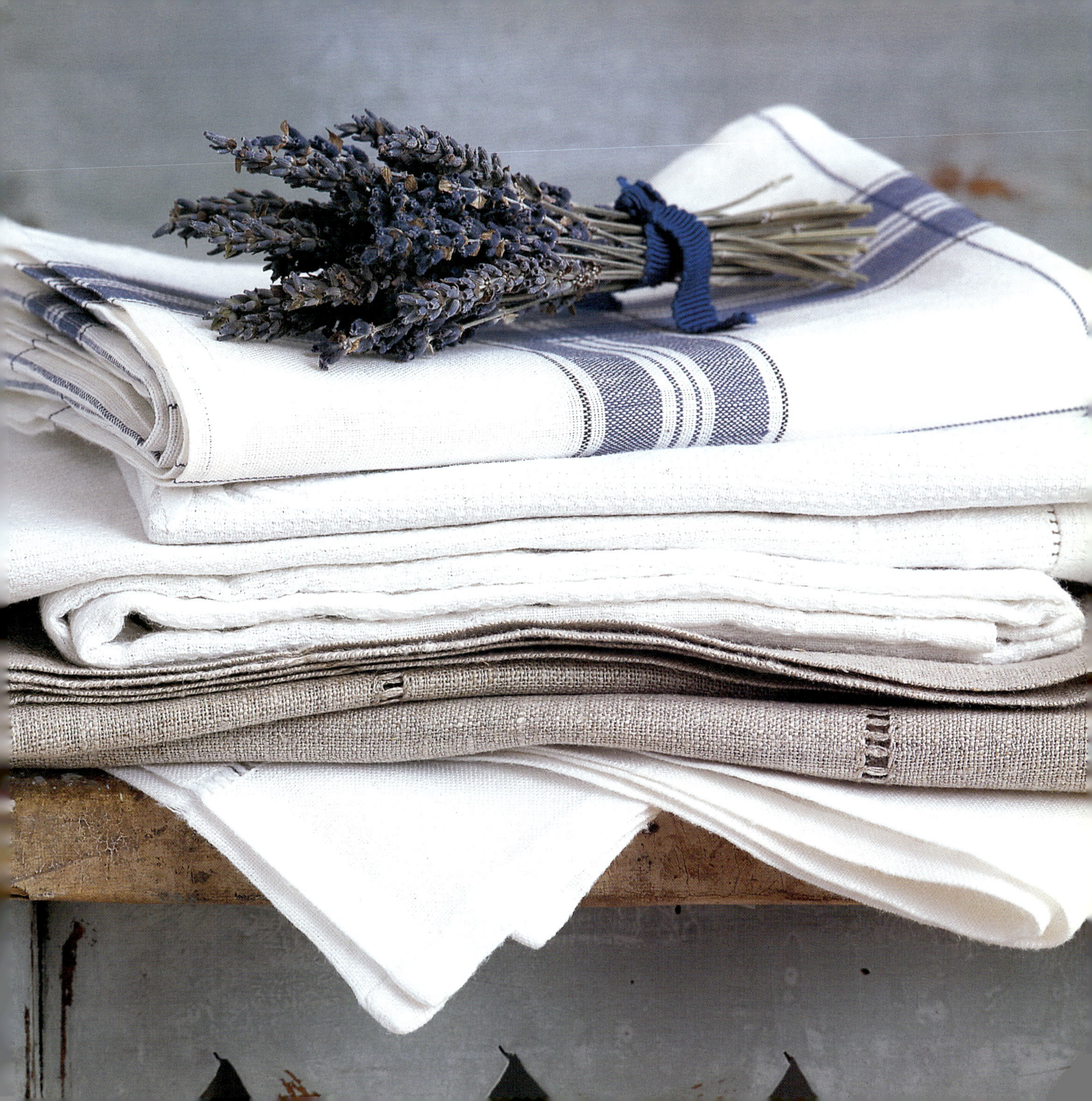

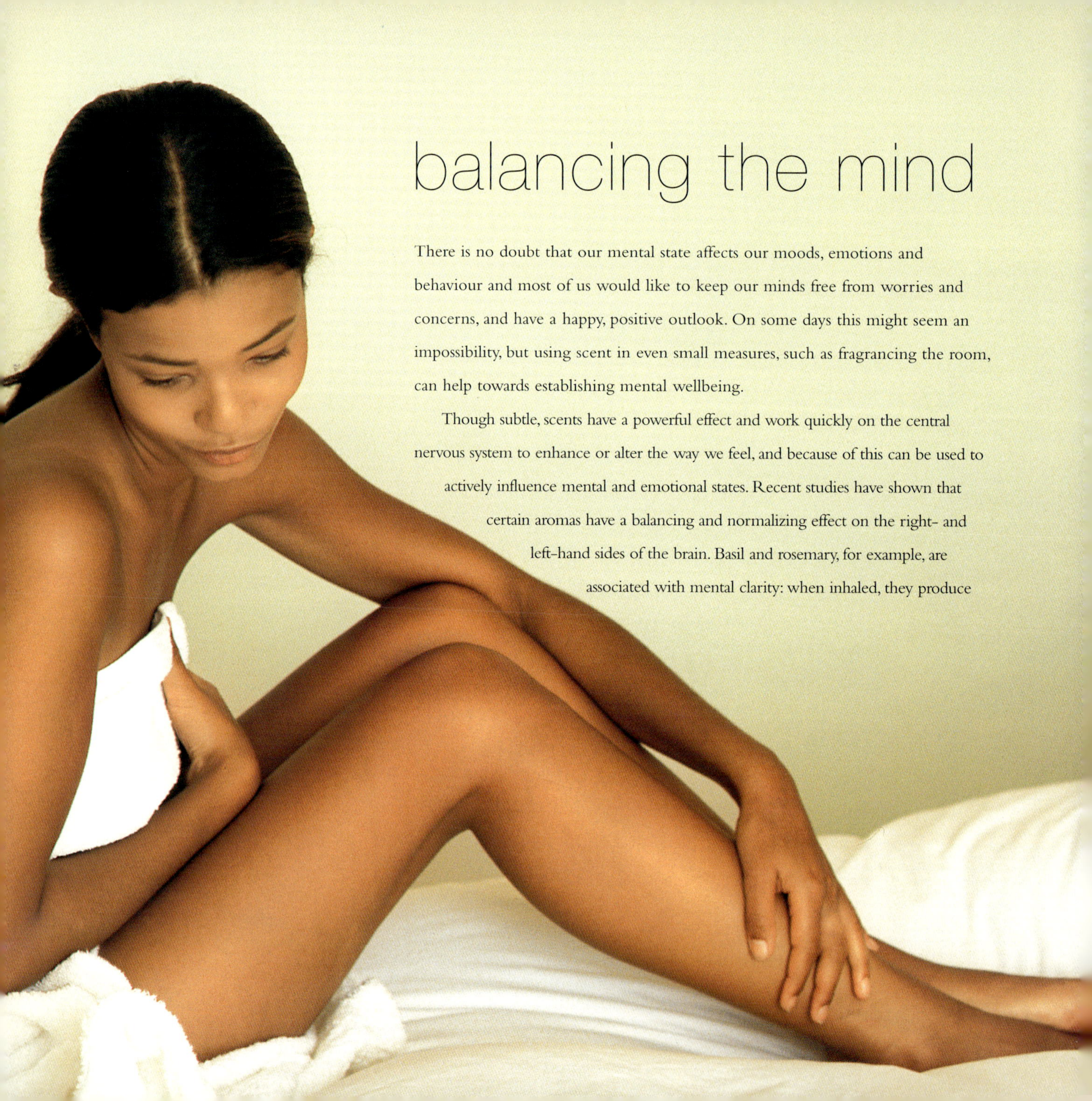

balancing the mind

There is no doubt that our mental state affects our moods, emotions and behaviour and most of us would like to keep our minds free from worries and concerns, and have a happy, positive outlook. On some days this might seem an impossibility, but using scent in even small measures, such as fragrancing the room, can help towards establishing mental wellbeing.

Though subtle, scents have a powerful effect and work quickly on the central nervous system to enhance or alter the way we feel, and because of this can be used to actively influence mental and emotional states. Recent studies have shown that certain aromas have a balancing and normalizing effect on the right- and left-hand sides of the brain. Basil and rosemary, for example, are associated with mental clarity: when inhaled, they produce a brain-rhythm pattern that shows alertness. Calming scents, such as rose, neroli and jasmine, on the other hand, induce relaxed rhythms, similar to those shown by the mind when approaching a state of meditation.

Achieving a relaxed, calm state of mind can be difficult in today's world. Stress and stress-related illnesses are on the increase, and we face mounting pressures in many areas of our lives: at work, at home, in our relationships, and with our children. It is hardly surprising that we feel overwhelmed and unable to cope sometimes.

Rose, neroli and jasmine induce calm, relaxed mind rhythms, similar to those produced by a state of meditation.

Using fragrance in our daily lives is one way of countering some of the negative effects of stress, depression, tension and anxiety. Scents can help us to relax and unwind, they can energize and fortify us, and they can help restore balance and harmony by ministering to our emotional and mental states. By cultivating the use of scent in our daily lives we can encourage and nurture a positive outlook.

Essential to using scents productively, however, is to discover what works best for yourself – both in the choice of scents and the method of introducing them into your lifestyle. Set aside some quiet time each day to relax, even if it is only for ten or fifteen minutes. On a summer day, sit outside and enjoy the smell of freshly mown grass, sweetly scented honeysuckle, or intoxicating lilac. If you are indoors, light a fragrant candle, vaporize an aromatic oil, or soak in a scented bath. The sense of smell is very individual so don't hesitate to explore new aromas – part of the pleasure of using scents is discovering favourite blends, which can only help in regaining your equilibrium.

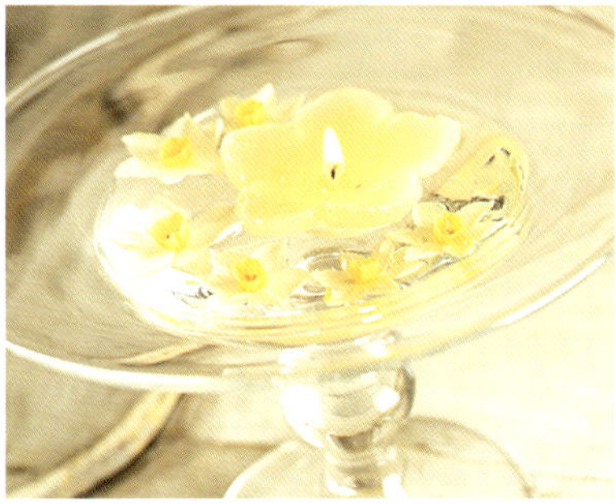

opposite Finding time for yourself can often be a cure in itself.
above Gently scented candles with rose or jasmine, surrounded by pretty flowers, can act as a simple reminder of the need for quiet moments.
below Essential oils, such as those from the basil plant, can promote clear thinking.

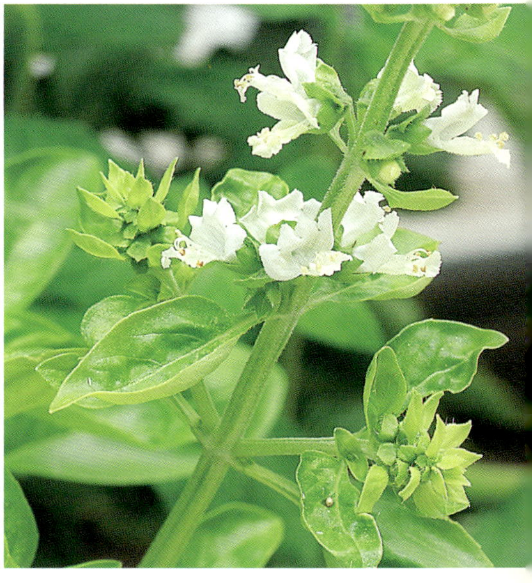

nourishing the body

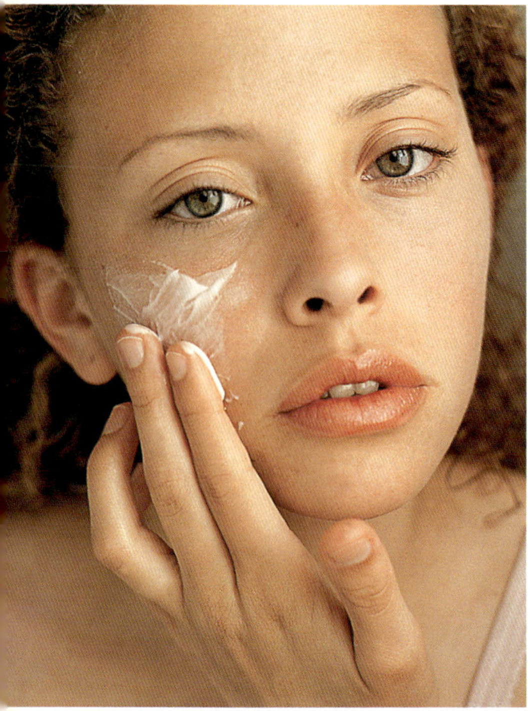

The body is sometimes referred to as "the temple of the soul" and in order to feel healthy and balanced we need to look after its needs. Some of these needs include adequate sleep, a balanced diet and taking regular exercise. Properly followed, these ground rules will help keep our bodies free from toxins, our immune system strong, and promote a blooming, clear complexion. In addition, we can use scent in our daily bodycare regime, with aromatic oils, lotions and creams on our skin, in massage and bathing to help us relax and sleep well, and in food and drink.

Most of us require around eight hours of sleep a night. It is during this time that our body's cells regenerate and renew themselves. If we have insufficient sleep or sleep of poor quality, our system never gets a chance to relax properly. A few drops of lavender on your pillow at bedtime may help if you have trouble sleeping.

You are what you eat is an old maxim, but it is still true. Without a healthy diet, our body's cells receive insufficient nutrition. A diet that is high in refined foods, sugar, alcohol and caffeine will put a strain on the body's systems as they struggle to function properly without the right nourishment. Try substituting peppermint tea for caffeine drinks, particularly if you suffer from digestive problems, or for a weakened immune system, eat foods containing aromatic herbs and spices, such as ginger and garlic, to give it a boost.

Most of us lead increasingly sedentary lifestyles, and we need to ensure we get sufficient exercise. Physical activity improves the circulation and promotes the elimination of toxins from the lymphatic system. A build up of toxins can lead to a variety of problems including cellulite and other imbalances in our body and skin. Use scents in massage to provide further help in eliminating toxins.

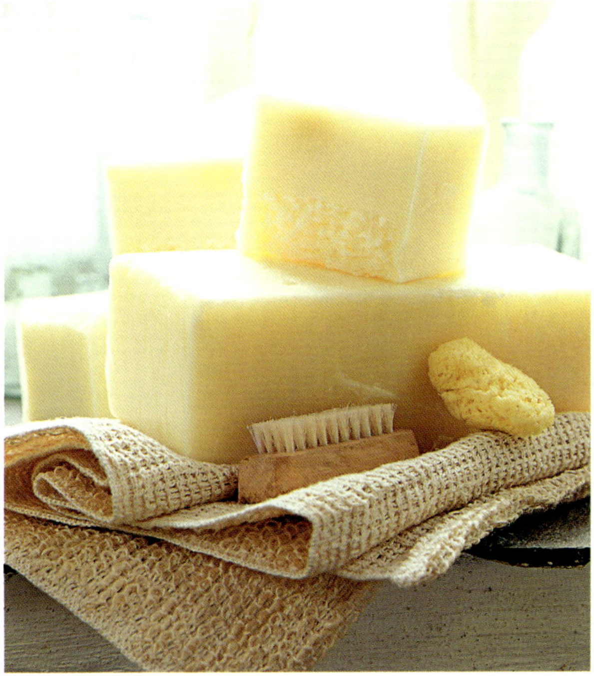

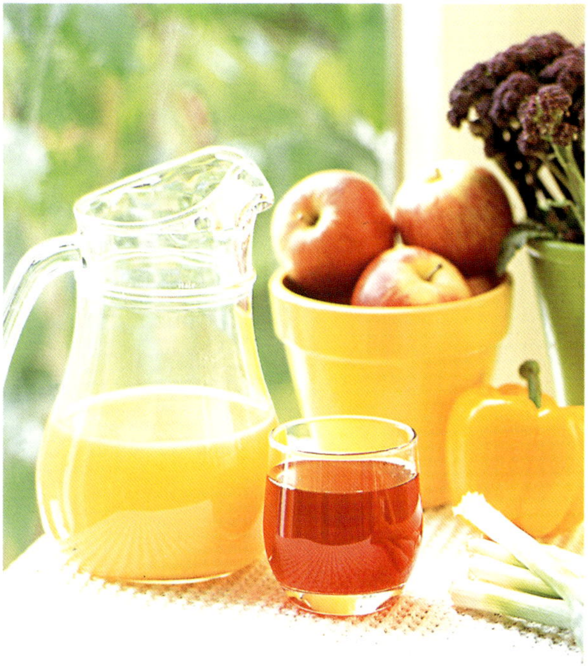

Looking after our skin is also important. The skin is the largest organ of the body and its condition is a good indicator of our general health. A skin problem can arise from many causes, such as poor digestion, or from a mental or emotional imbalance, such as deep-rooted anxiety or grief. Establishing a skincare regime which cleanses, tones and moisturizes will help preserve the healthy appearance of our skin. Rather than considering such attention a chore, this is an area where scented products really come into their own, and the opportunities for pampering ourselves with sweetly-smelling oils, creams and lotions are endless. Body products containing rose, jasmine, lavender and sandalwood are particularly beneficial.

opposite Treat and nourish your skin using scented creams and lotions.
above left Handmade soaps may not last as long as the average bar of commercially produced soap, but they are lovely as a special treat and make wonderful bath companions.
above right A healthy diet is one which contains plenty of fresh fruit and vegetables. Try and drink water and vegetable or fruit juices rather than tea or coffee.

reviving the spirit

Many people believe that a strong and healthy connection with the inner self is the way to happiness, and that disease actually originates with a departure from our inner spirituality.

In today's world it is very easy to lose touch with ourselves and to feel out of sorts. We are so often preoccupied and busy that we are unable to hear the "still small voice of the soul" or our intuition that is trying to communicate with us and guide us in the right direction.

Around the world, fragrance has a long tradition of use in religious ceremonies as an aid to meditation and reflection, and certain aromas have the power to transform mundane mental states into higher, more meditative levels of consciousness. Sandalwood incense is burned in Hindu temples for example, frankincense is used in the Roman Catholic mass, and sprigs of fresh juniper are burned in Tibetan temples as a form of healing and purification.

The ancient Chinese believed that by extracting a plant's oils they were liberating its soul, and alchemists strove to find the elixir of eternal life in these "magical" essences.

In much the same way that we need to look after our bodies with the right diet, adequate sleep and plenty of fresh air and exercise, it is important to nourish our inner selves. There are many ways in which we can do this and it is a question of each individual finding a method that works. Walking outdoors, spending time alone, enjoying creative pursuits, making time for relationships, and setting aside quiet time for reflection are some of the ways in which we can take care of the spirit. Additionally, we can use scent to successfully build and maintain a connection with our spiritual selves.

Even if our reasons for doing so are less exalted, we can nevertheless still use fragrance as a way of reviving our flagging spirits. Whether we choose to burn incense during meditation, light a perfumed candle as we take a bath or enjoy sweetly scented flowers in our living room, we are using fragrance to lift our spirits and bring us back into balance and harmony.

opposite For days when even the ordinary activities of life seem too difficult, a room of one's own to retreat to is essential: create a haven for yourself with scented fabrics and gentle lighting, perfume the air with calming and soothing fragrances of your choice, and relax.

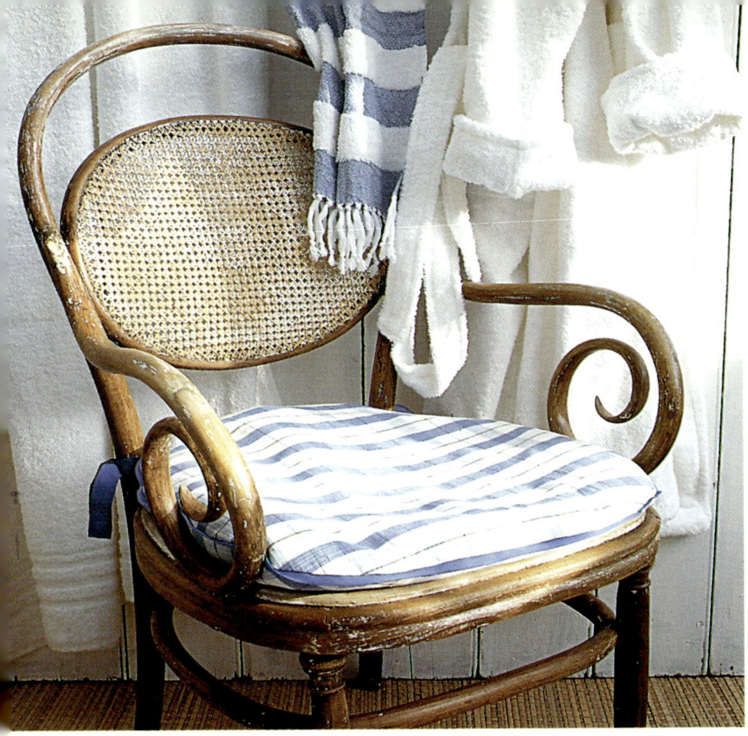
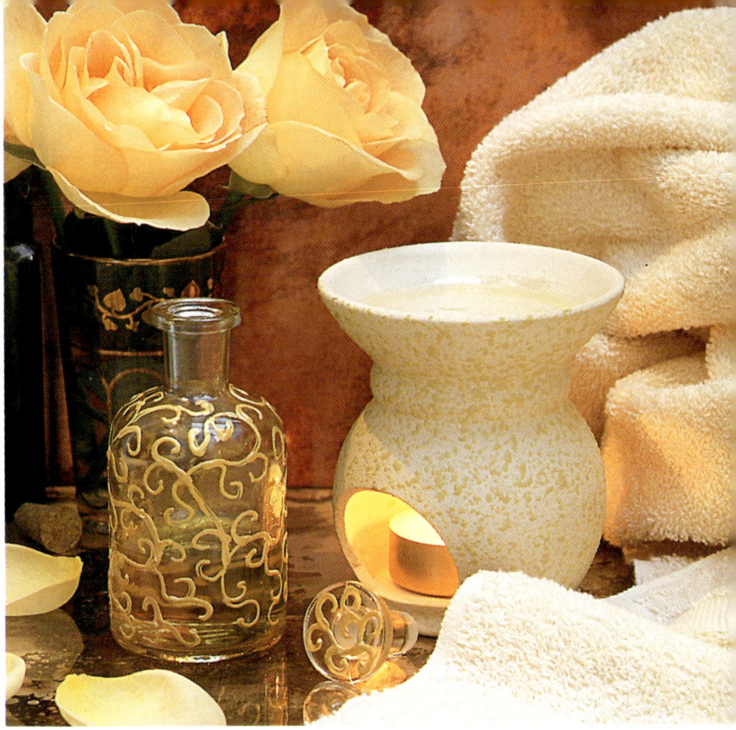
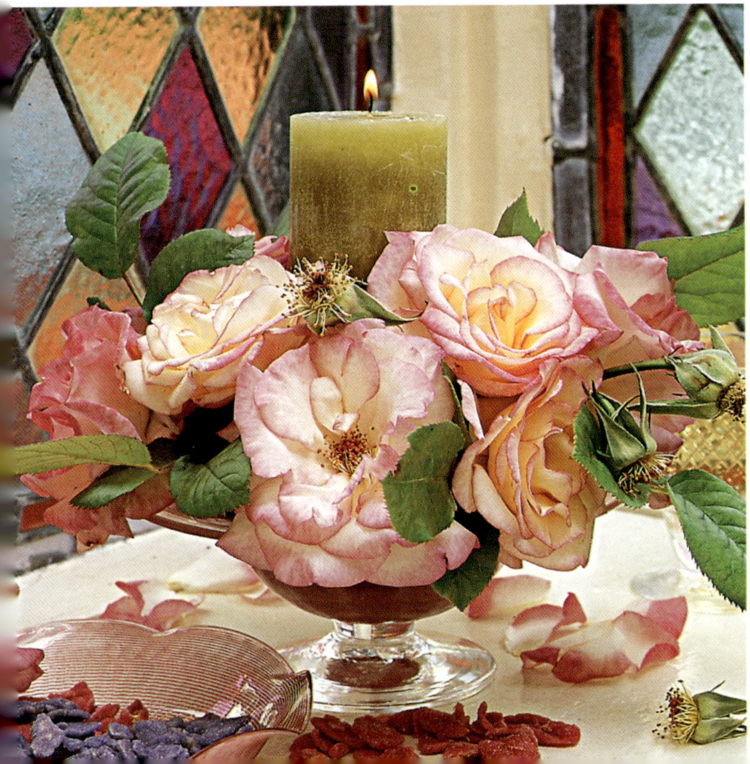
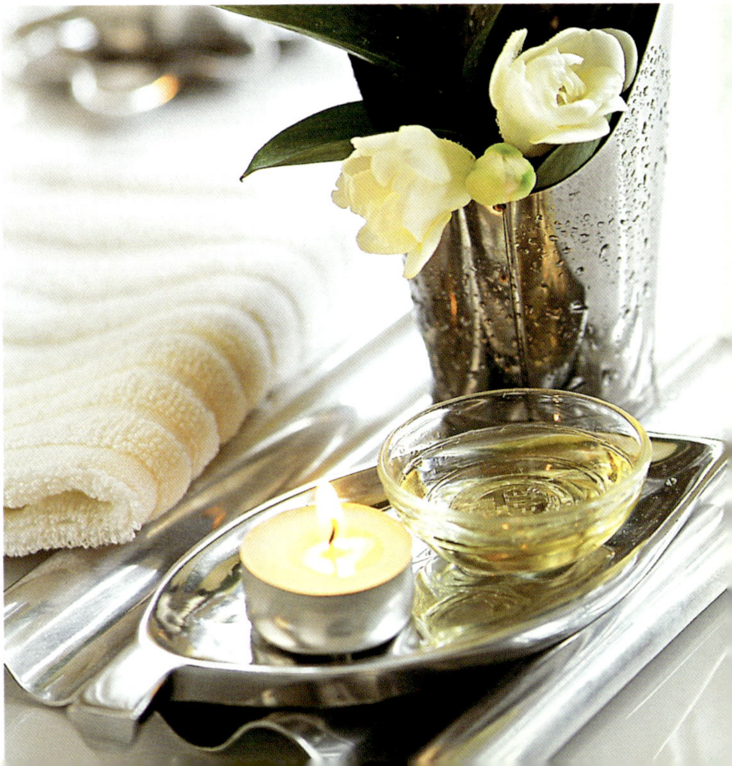

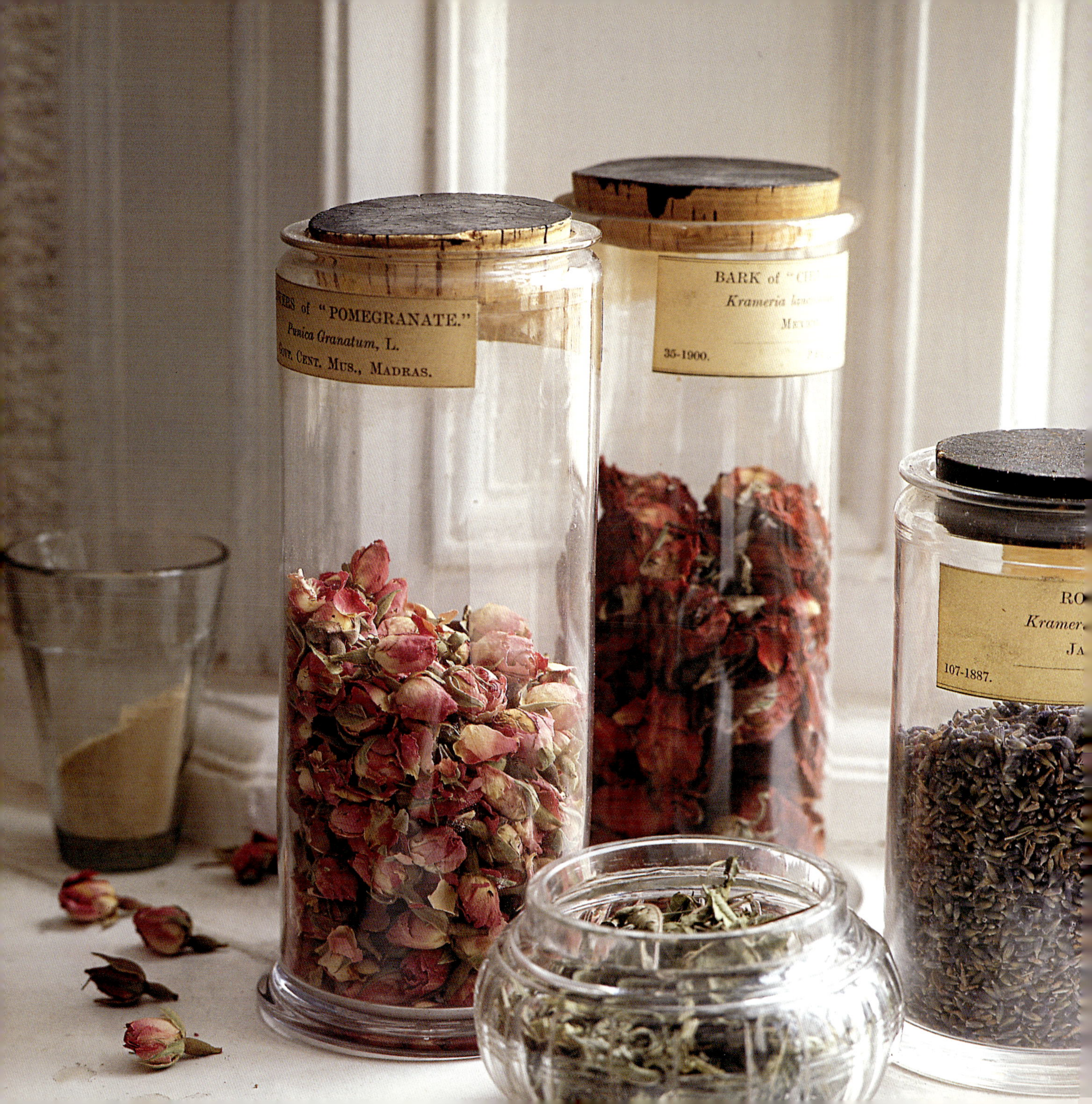

of "POMEGRANATE."
Punica Granatum, L.
Cent. Mus., Madras.
BARK of
Krameria
35-1900.
107-1887.

a potpourri of aromas

When first learning about scents and their therapeutic properties, the sheer range of aromas can seem bewildering, and it's difficult to know how to match need with scent. The following pages helps you to do just that, by offering plenty of suggestions for dealing with the ups and downs of life – for example, if you are in need of a burst of energy for an important meeting, there are ideas on using scents to invigorate or stimulate. Or, if you are seeking a good night's sleep, there are tips on how to use scents to help you relax and unwind at the end of the day. Discover, too, how all parts of the aromatic plant from fresh flowers to fragrant spices can be used easily and effectively.

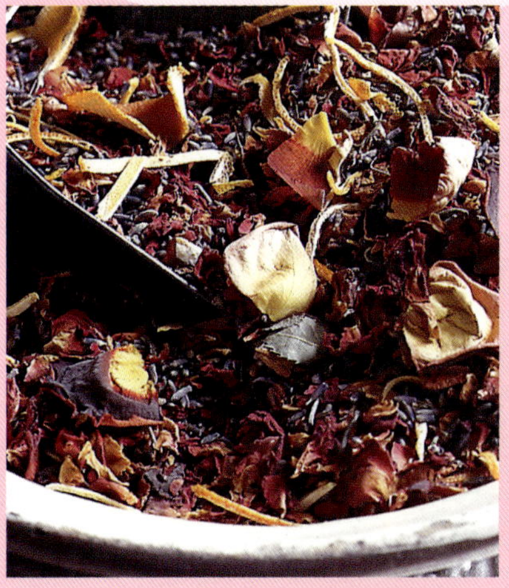

invigorating

When we are feeling tired and sluggish, fresh and spicy aromas will give us a helpful boost. Ginger, coriander and black pepper are three powerful stimulants, which can either be included in your daily diet or added to bath oils, lotions and muscle rubs. They should be used with restraint, however: ginger and black pepper may irritate sensitive skins.

Fiery ginger, which is used in Chinese medicine for its stimulating properties, warms and brings life to the body, and is especially beneficial for the circulation – sufferers of cold hands and feet should add a few drops of the essential oil to a vegetable base oil to help dilute and spread it, and rub it on to the affected areas each day.

Coriander (cilantro) was also well known to the ancient Chinese who believed its seeds contained the power of immortality. This herb has a fresh and spicy aroma and is useful when you are feeling drained or sluggish.

One of the earliest known spices, black pepper, has been prized throughout history. Attila the Hun reputedly demanded more than a ton of it as part of the ransom for Rome. Its warming effect makes it an ideal muscle rub, particularly before exercise. Combined with rosemary, black pepper essential oil has been used by athletes to achieve faster times and to reduce muscular fatigue and pain. Try it yourself before a workout.

Coriander, ginger and black pepper are also effective aphrodisiacs, particularly for men. One source cites that the women of Senegal weave ginger root into their husband's belts to arouse their sexual interest.

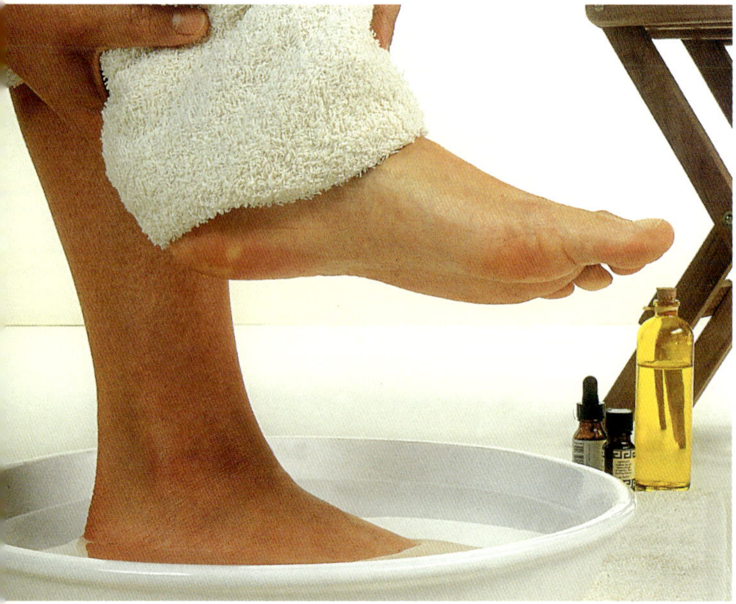

left Use ginger essential oil in footbaths to stimulate the circulation.
opposite Add spice to recipes with scented vinegars and oils, such as this vibrant chilli and black peppercorn vinegar or this delicious coriander olive oil.
opposite right The whole foot will benefit from a massage with a lotion containing essential oils. Use sweeping motions to aid circulation.

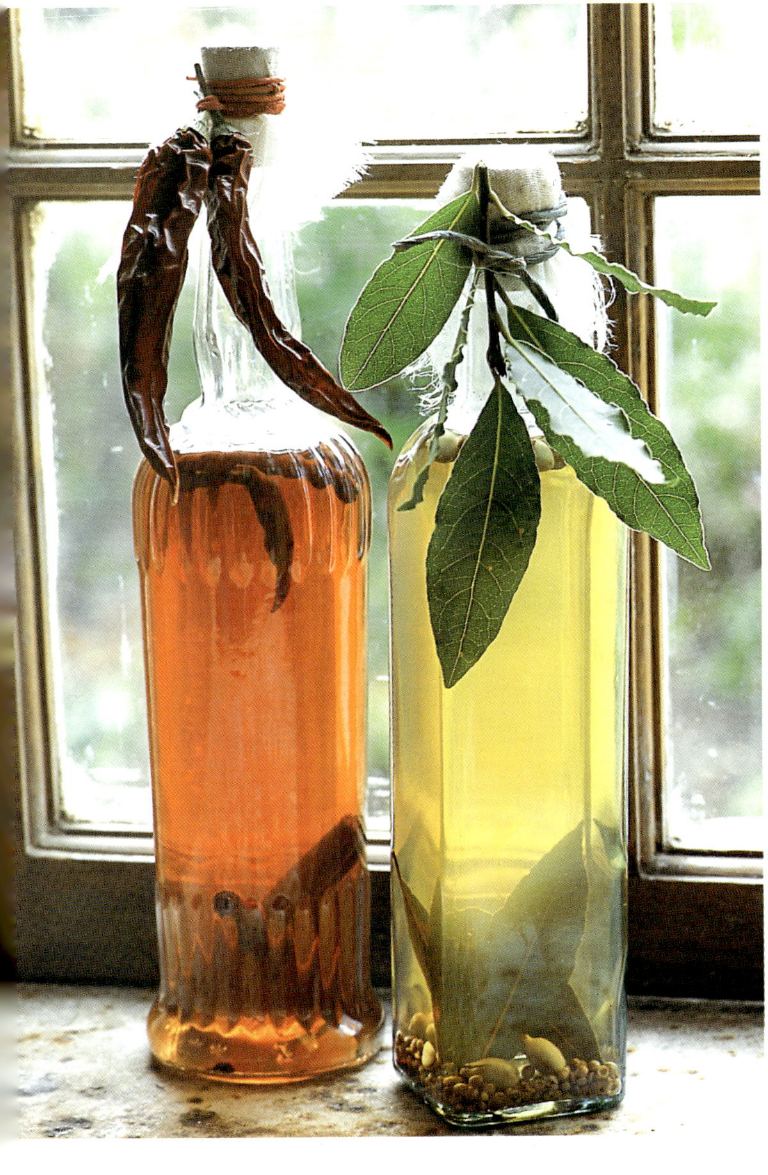

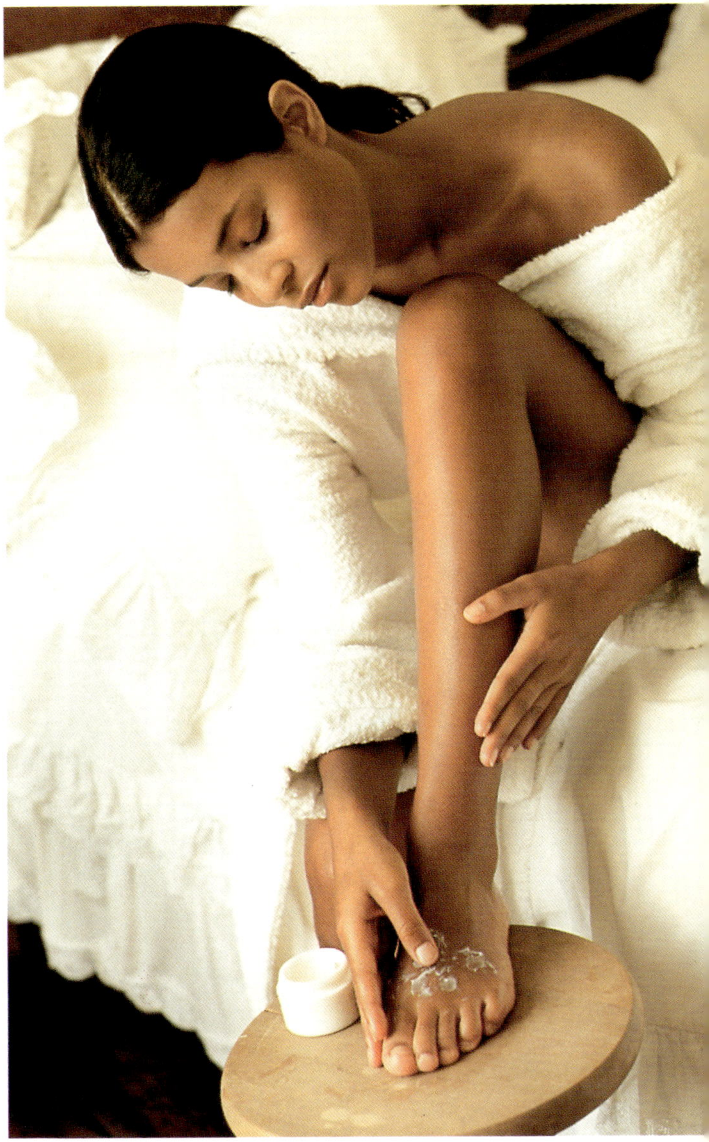

stimulating

Mental fatigue calls for scents that will blow away the cobwebs, clearing away confusion and indecision, and restoring clarity and a positive outlook.

The clear, invigorating vapour of fresh rosemary is a wonderful stimulant to mental clarity; a fact known to students in ancient Greece, who wore sprigs of the fresh herb in their hair to improve their memory. Peppermint was another scent widely appreciated by the ancient Greeks, as well as the Egyptians, Chinese and Indians. The Romans used to crown themselves with peppermint wreaths during lavish feasts, in order to take advantage of its detoxifying effects. Today, scents in the form of essential oils are used in many stimulating ways.

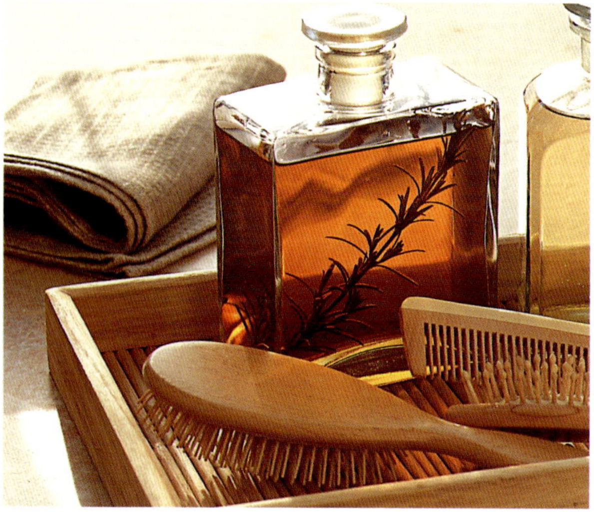

above Rosemary is renowned for its ability to restore shine to hair that is dull and lifeless: try adding several drops of the essential oil to an unscented shampoo base, or make up your own shampoo with whole sprigs of rosemary.

Peppermint essential oil is excellent when used as an inhalant or mixed with a base cream and rubbed on to the temples. Its clear, minty smell will open the sinuses and relieve tension headaches. Both rosemary and peppermint help promote inspiration and insight. Their scents will clear your head and pep up your brain cells – ideal for situations where alertness is essential. To relieve tiredness, such as when on long journeys, add a few drops of each fragrance to a mist sprayer to spritz over your face at intervals.

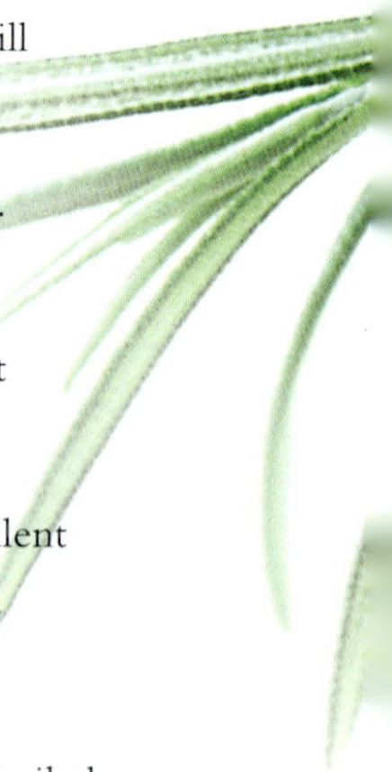

Similarly, the fresh, pungent smell of basil is excellent for relieving mental fatigue; during the 16th century it was ground into a powder and inhaled like snuff to clear headaches, head colds and blocked sinuses. Basil also helps to recharge the memory, and so is ideal for aiding concentration. If you need to start your day feeling more alert than usual, add a few drops to a morning bath to wake up your system and give you extra energy.

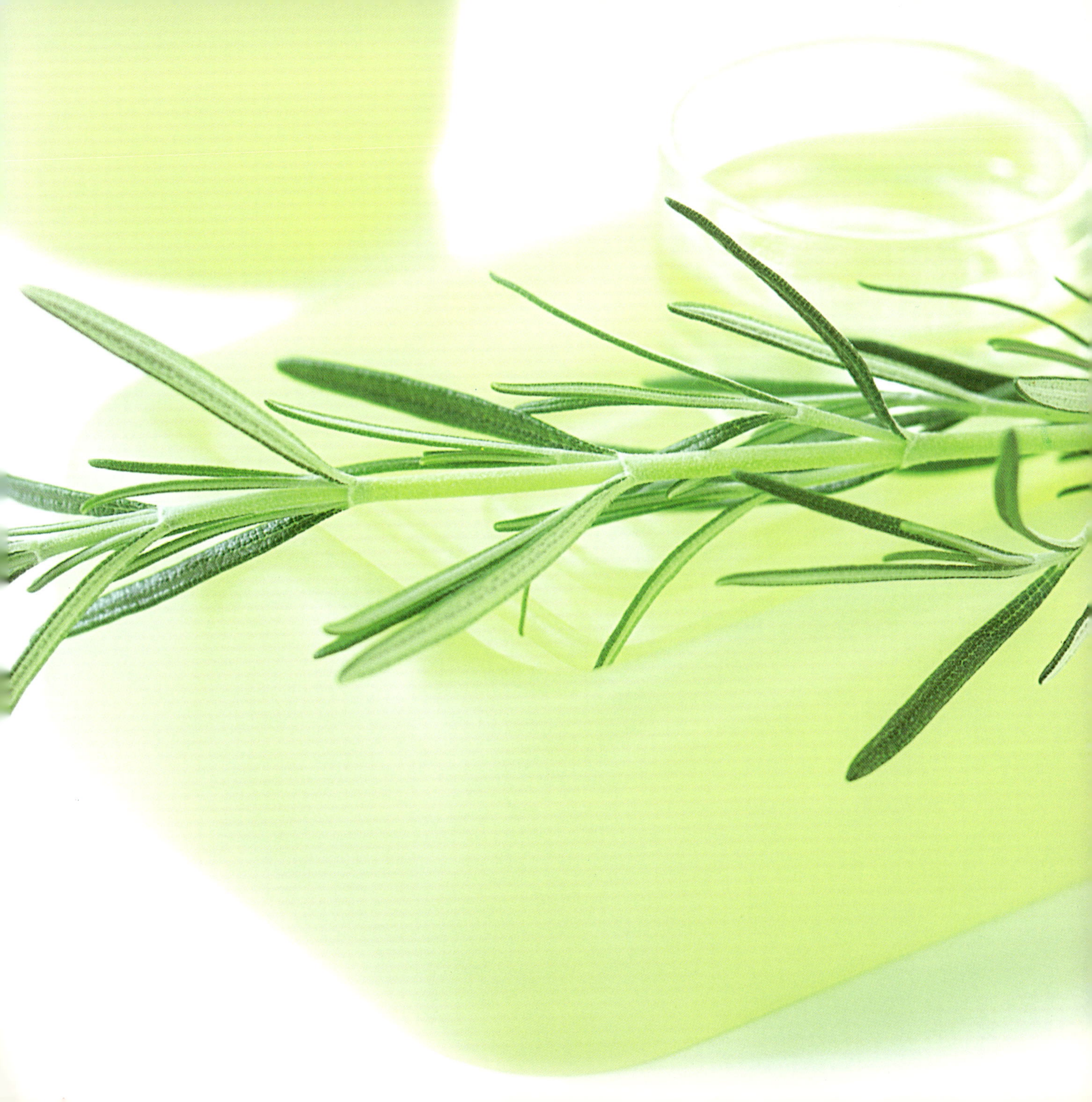

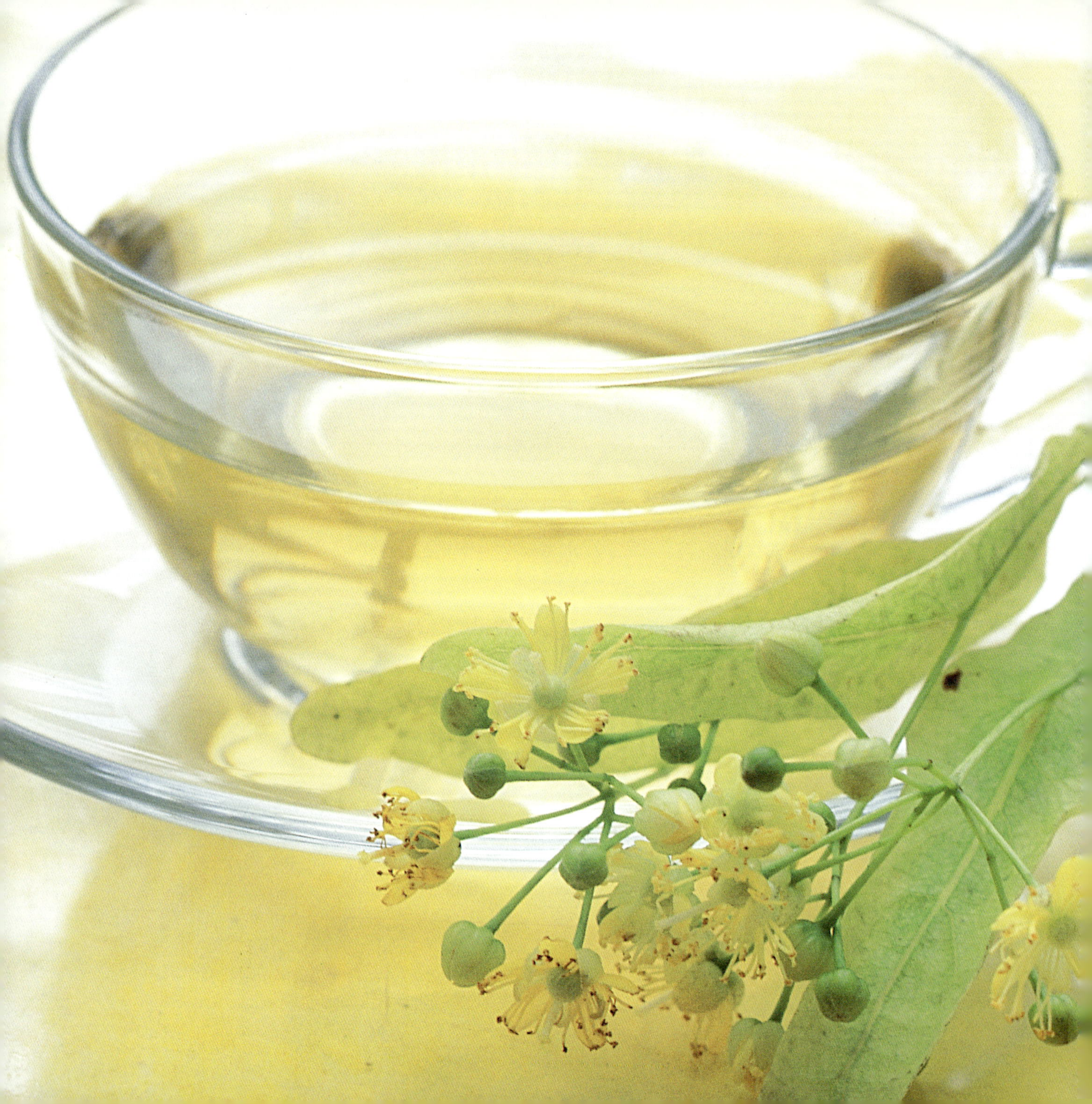

refreshing

Citrus fragrances are the first ones to look for when you are seeking an uplifting and cooling effect. Their aromas are light and zingy, and they have healing and cleansing properties. Lime, lemon and grapefruit are all sharp and refreshing, ideal when you are feeling hot, tired and drained of energy.

opposite Soothing lime blossom tea.
below In addition to their aromatic leaves, many herbs have beautiful flowers. Bergamot flowers range from bright pink, red, and purple to white.

When your spirits are flagging, drink a revitalizing cup of tea; Earl Grey tea will both refresh and cleanse.

Possibly the most cleansing of the citrus oils, lemon sharpens the mind and dispels confusion. In a room spray, it gives a clean, fresh, harmonizing aroma. Lime is good for nervous exhaustion and stress-related disorders and grapefruit awakens the spirits; it is useful when feeling lethargic and low.

As well as bearing cheerful bright flowers, bergamot has a light citrus aroma and is useful as a room freshener, eliminating stale, musty odours and cooking smells. When your spirits are flagging, there is no easier remedy than a refreshing cup of Earl Grey tea, which gets its distinctive aroma and taste from bergamot essential oil.

Alternatively, opt for the clean, woody aromas of a shady evergreen forest. The scent of pine is strong, dry and balsamic; its effect is refreshing, cooling and enlivening. Pine is helpful with excessive perspiration, fatigue and stress-related disorders. Cypress also has a fresh balsamic odour and its effect is cooling and calming. The essential oil blends well with bergamot and other citrus essences.

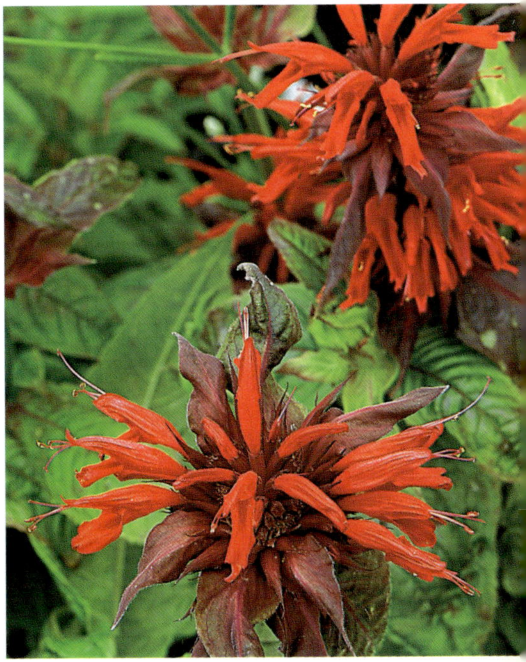

hair and skin zingers

Nowadays, there are many highly sophisticated products available for sale that will make your hair and skin glow, but far simpler, natural treatments can easily achieve the same results. Refreshing scents, such as lemon, grapefruit and cypress, have antiseptic and astringent properties, which make them ideal for treating greasy hair and oily skin problems.

If your hair is dull, lank and oily, add a few drops of grapefruit oil to an unperfumed shampoo base and use every second day. The result will be beautifully shiny, fragrant hair.

For hair that needs frequent washing don't be tempted to use harsh degreasing shampoos or to shampoo too often – the rubbing action on the scalp stimulates the sebaceous glands to produce more sebum, thus worsening the problem.

If you have oily or combination skin, pay attention to your diet and drink plenty of water. It also helps to adopt a good skincare regime as open pores easily become clogged with dirt, causing blackheads, spots and pimples. For a clear, healthy skin, add a few drops of lemon and lime oils to an unperfumed cream base and cleanse twice a day. Tone the skin with a sprizter containing refreshing scents such as orange, grapefruit and cypress.

opposite Make skincare part of your daily routine with a zesty, exfoliating citrus scrub.

citrus face and body scrub

Orange peel is mixed with the slightly gritty texture of ground sunflower seeds, oatmeal and sea salt in this reviving scrub, helping to remove dead skin cells and stimulate the blood supply to the skin, leaving it feeling tingling and toned. The combination of aromatic orange peel and refreshing grapefruit oil gives it a lovely clean scent.

you will need:
45ml/3 tbsp freshly ground sunflower seeds
45ml/3 tbsp medium oatmeal
45ml/3 tbsp flaked sea salt
45ml/3 tbsp finely grated orange peel
3 drops of grapefruit essential oil
almond oil

Mix together well all the ingredients except the almond oil and store in a sealed glass jar. Using just a little at a time, mix with some almond oil to make a thick paste, then rub over the face and body, paying particular attention to areas of dry skin such as the elbows, knees and ankles. Wipe off any residue with a tissue before showering or bathing.

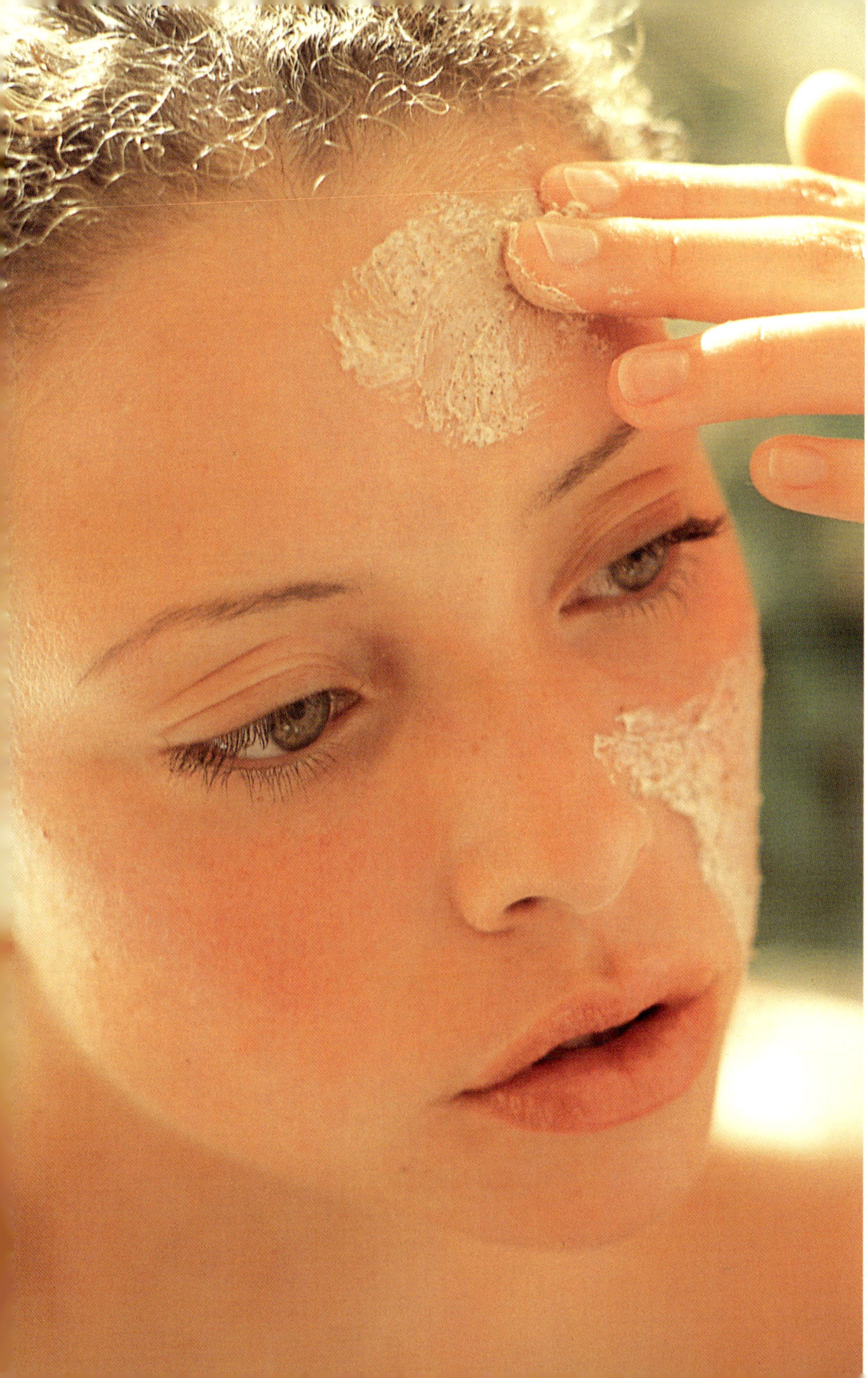
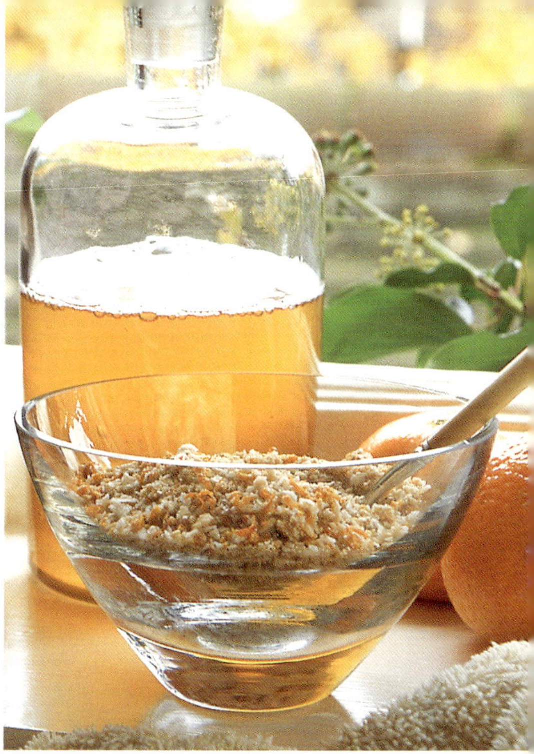
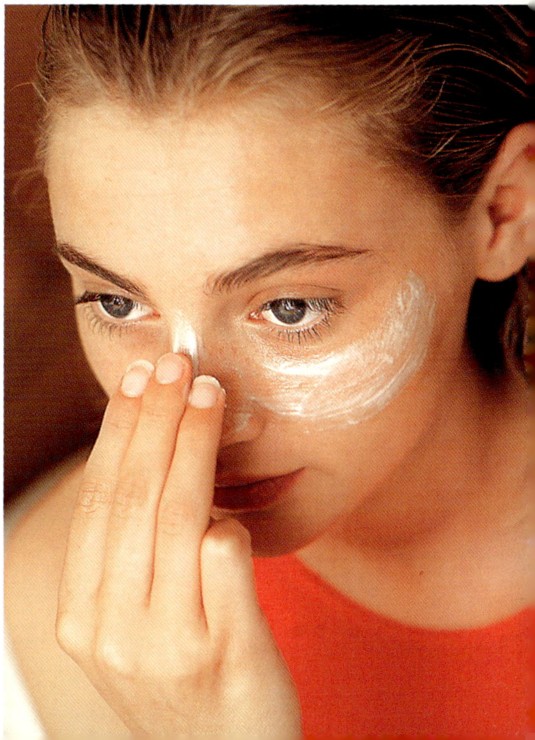

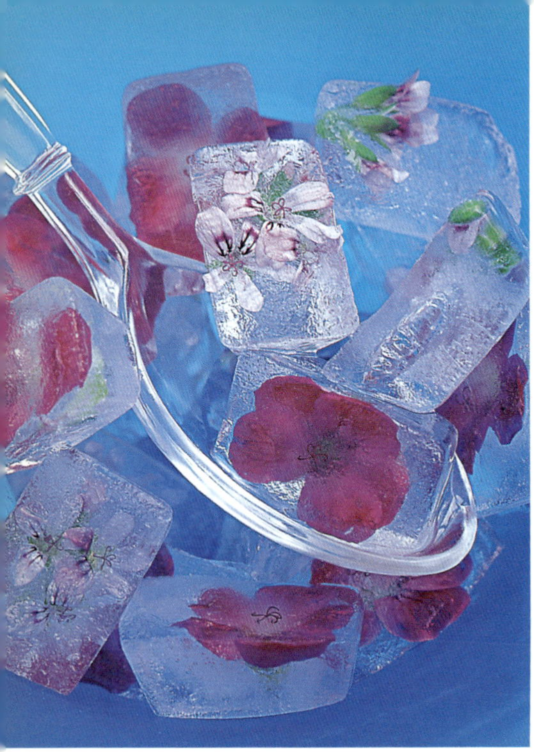

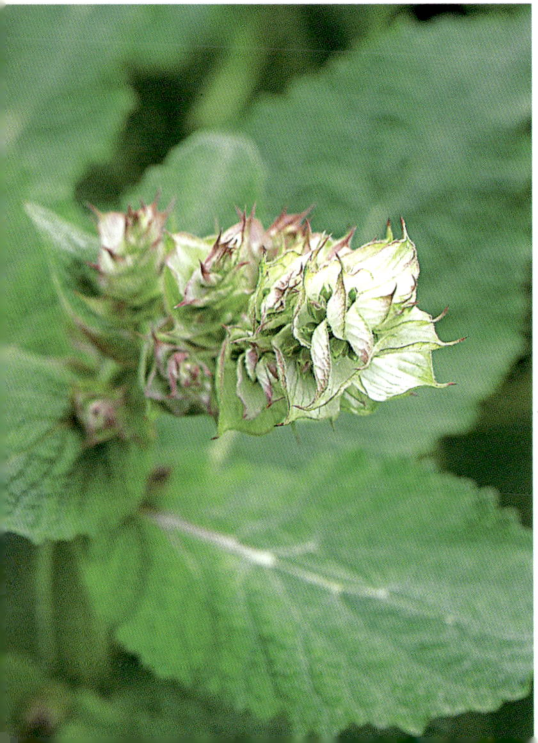

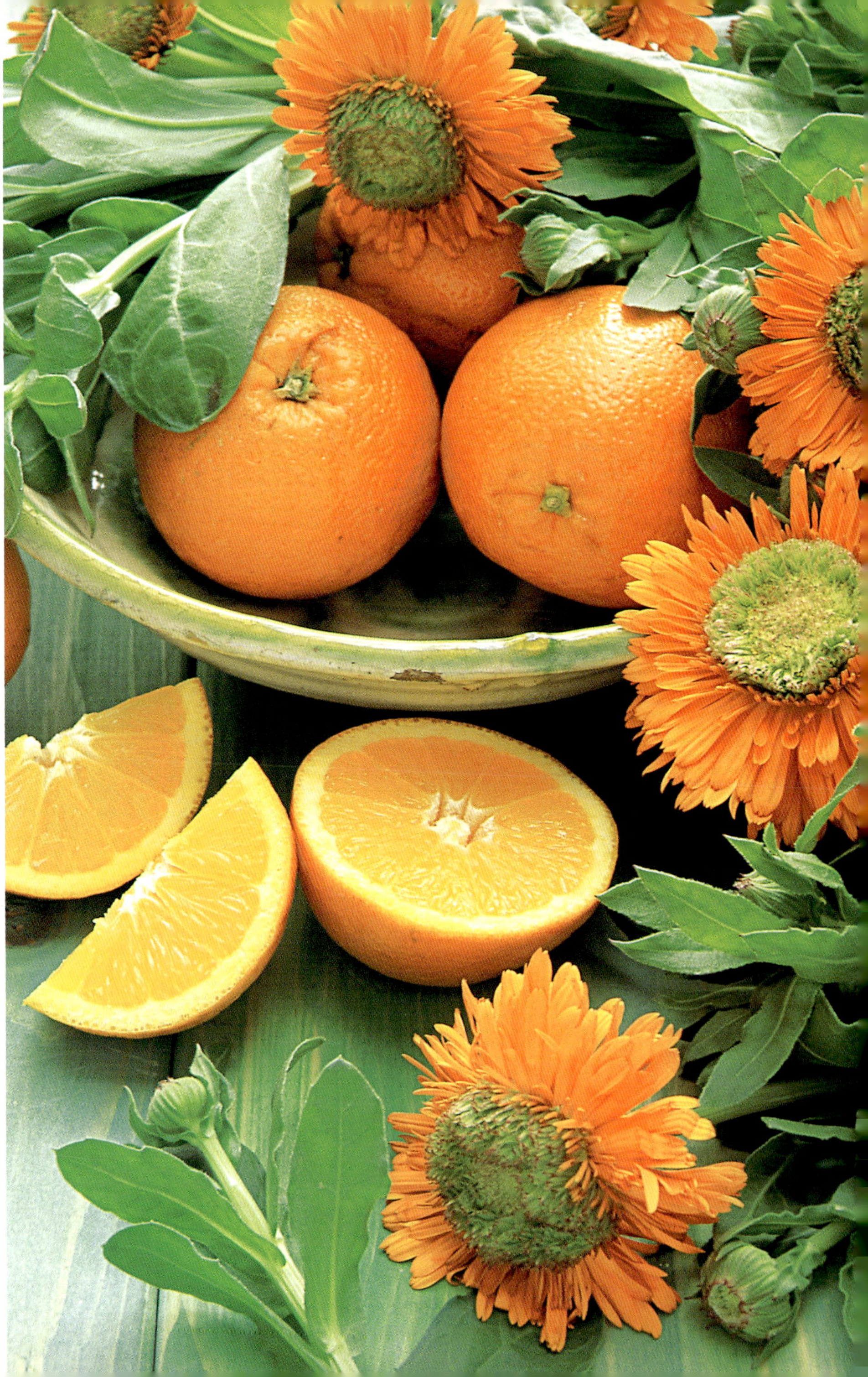

uplifting

When you are feeling blue and out of sorts, or are caught by worries and feelings of insecurity, look for fragrances that will lift your spirits and encourage a cheerful outlook.

The sweetly herbaceous, heady fragrance of clary sage will achieve a definite euphoric lift. If you are suffering from stress and nervous tension, try burning a few drops of the essential oil in a room vaporizer, but don't use too much, as you could be left feeling very light-headed.

The aroma of clary sage is also cleansing and it blends well with the sweet, refreshing aroma of orange, creating a cheering and uplifting combination. In China, gifts of oranges are offered during the New Year celebrations as symbols of happiness and prosperity. Their fresh aroma helps disperse gloomy, negative thoughts, revive the spirit and untangle emotional problems and obsessions.

The light, lemony scent of melissa is also reputed to chase away dark thoughts. A pleasant fragrance to have around the house or office, it encourages a clean and positive atmosphere. For depression associated with grief and loss, melissa will help bring understanding and relief.

The popular household plant, geranium, is another refreshing antidepressant, good for easing nervous tension and exhaustion and restoring harmony and balance. In Victorian Britain, the geranium plant was strategically placed around the house so that women's long skirts would brush against them and release the sweet and rosy perfume. For a refreshing, uplifting start to the day, blend two drops of geranium and two drops of bergamot essential oils and add to your bath just before you get in.

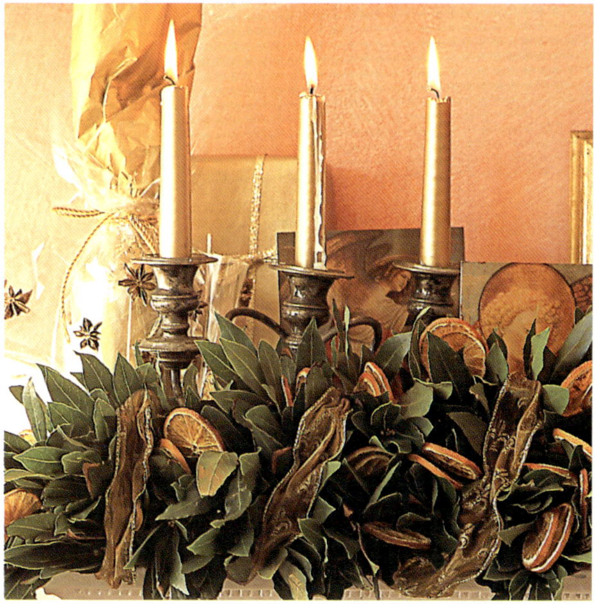

opposite Uplifting scents in the home and garden can have a powerful, uplifting effect on our moods.
above The warm tones of ried orange slices nestling in glossy evergreen bay leaves make a wonderfully aromatic Christmas garland.

calming and strengthening

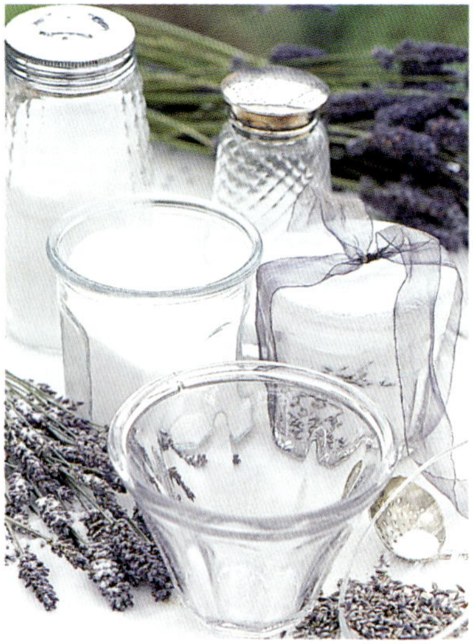

above Sugar scented with dried lavender flowers will add an exotic aroma to sweet recipes.
opposite Add chamomile flowers to bath oil for a pretty, and beneficial, effect.

Everyday life is full of pressures and it is easy to feel stressed, irritable and out of control. When our nerves are on edge, our immune system is weakened and we are more likely to succumb to infection or to suffer from stress-related disorders.

Lavender is one of nature's greatest "cure-alls" – it's a soothing tonic for the nervous system, capable of calming stormy emotional states and rebalancing the mind and body. If you suffer from tension headaches, try rubbing lavender oil on to the temples, or you could try an old remedy – Queen Elizabeth I of England drank copious cups of lavender tea to treat her frequent migraine headaches.

Chamomile is also known for its gentle, soothing properties. The ancient Egyptians dedicated the chamomile plant to the sun because of its ability to reduce feverish conditions. This gentle yet strengthening herb is particularly useful in treating inflammatory disorders of the digestive tract and sensitive skin conditions, such as eczema, which are often linked to tension and anxiety. Try adding a few drops to a base oil and using in massage and hot compresses.

The delicate fragrant flowers of the Seville orange tree produce a bitter-sweet oil, neroli, that is especially valuable for easing anxiety. Neroli helps to promote confidence in stressful situations: to calm jittery nerves before an engagement, or to cope with public speaking or interview nerves, take a handkerchief sprinkled with a few drops of neroli, and sniff it beforehand.

Sweet marjoram also calms nervous tension and has a strong sedative action. It can be comforting in times of grief, and its warm and woody aroma makes it particularly appealing to men who have trouble sleeping – use judiciously, however, because it is also reputed to quell sexual desire.

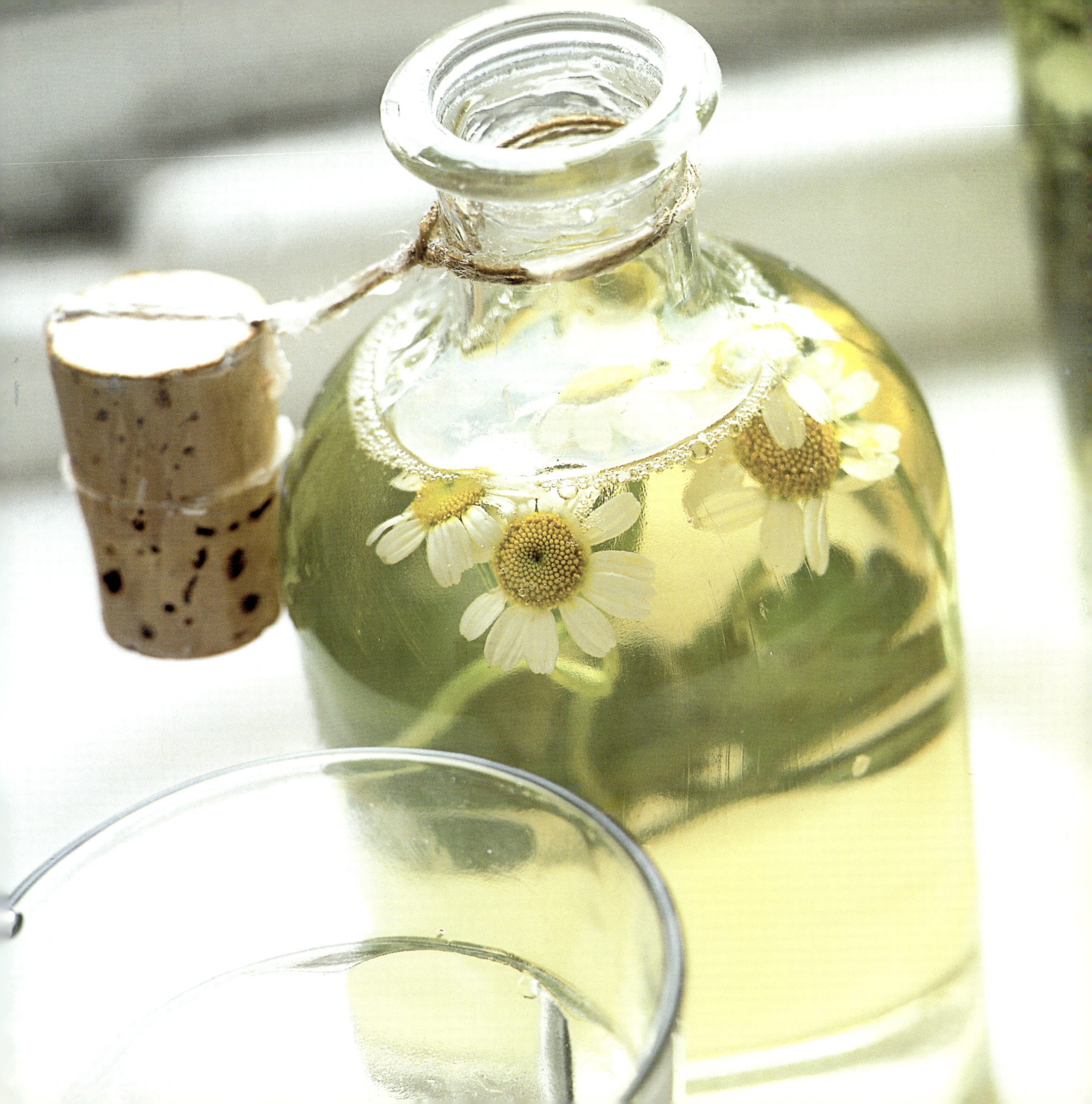

soothing slumbers

We have all experienced sleepless nights from time to time – worries go round and round inside our heads, just as we are trying to get to sleep. The resulting disturbed and restless night leaves us more prone to stress and anxiety, and a vicious cycle can be created. You can help break this cycle by taking a warm and fragrant bath at bedtime.

Bath salts have traditionally been used as a treatment for a variety of complaints, including skin problems and rheumatic aches and pains. If you have problems sleeping, treat yourself by making the following special blend. It will relax a tired mind and ease aching muscles, encouraging a good night's sleep.

goodnight bath salts

Chamomile is a widely recognized sedative; for these bath salts it has been combined with sweet marjoram, which is an effective treatment for insomnia.

you will need:
500g/1¼lb coarse sea salt
10 drops of chamomile essential oil
10 drops of sweet marjoram essential oil
1–3 drops of green food colouring (optional)

Combine all the ingredients and pour into a glass storage jar, with a close-fitting lid. Put the lid on firmly. Just before bedtime, light a scented candle, add a handful of the salts to your bath, immerse yourself in the warm water, and relax.

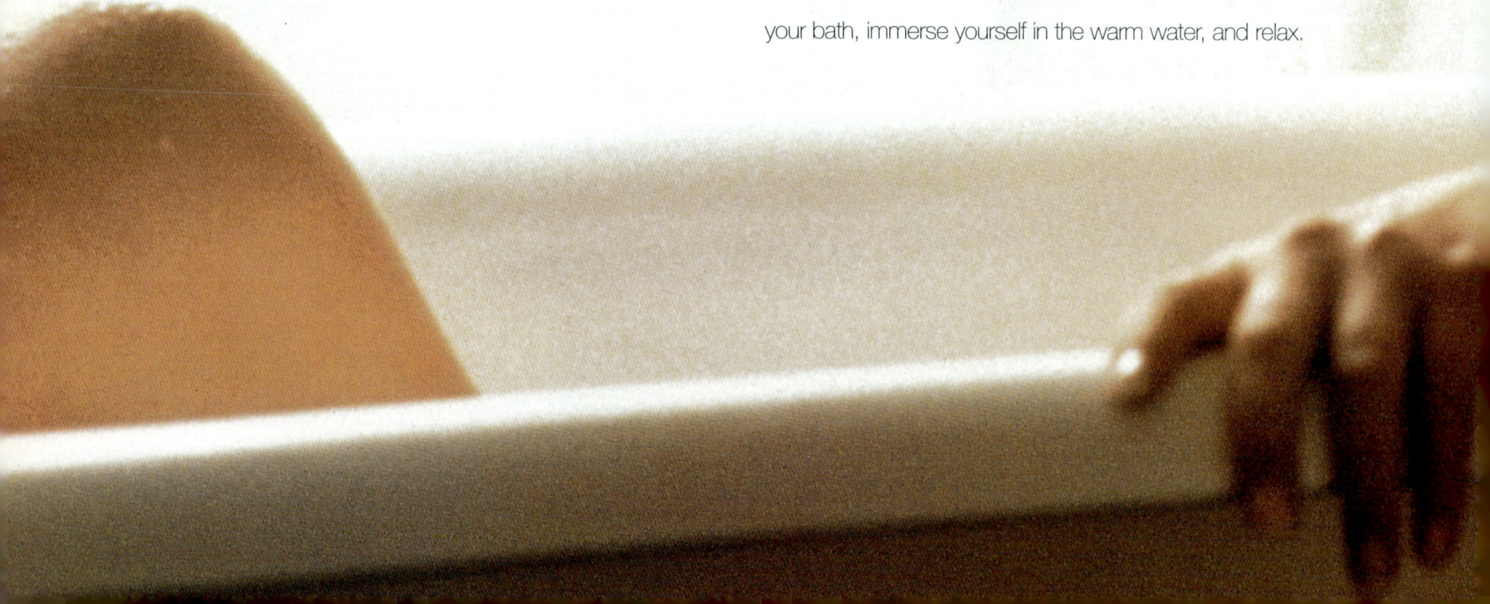

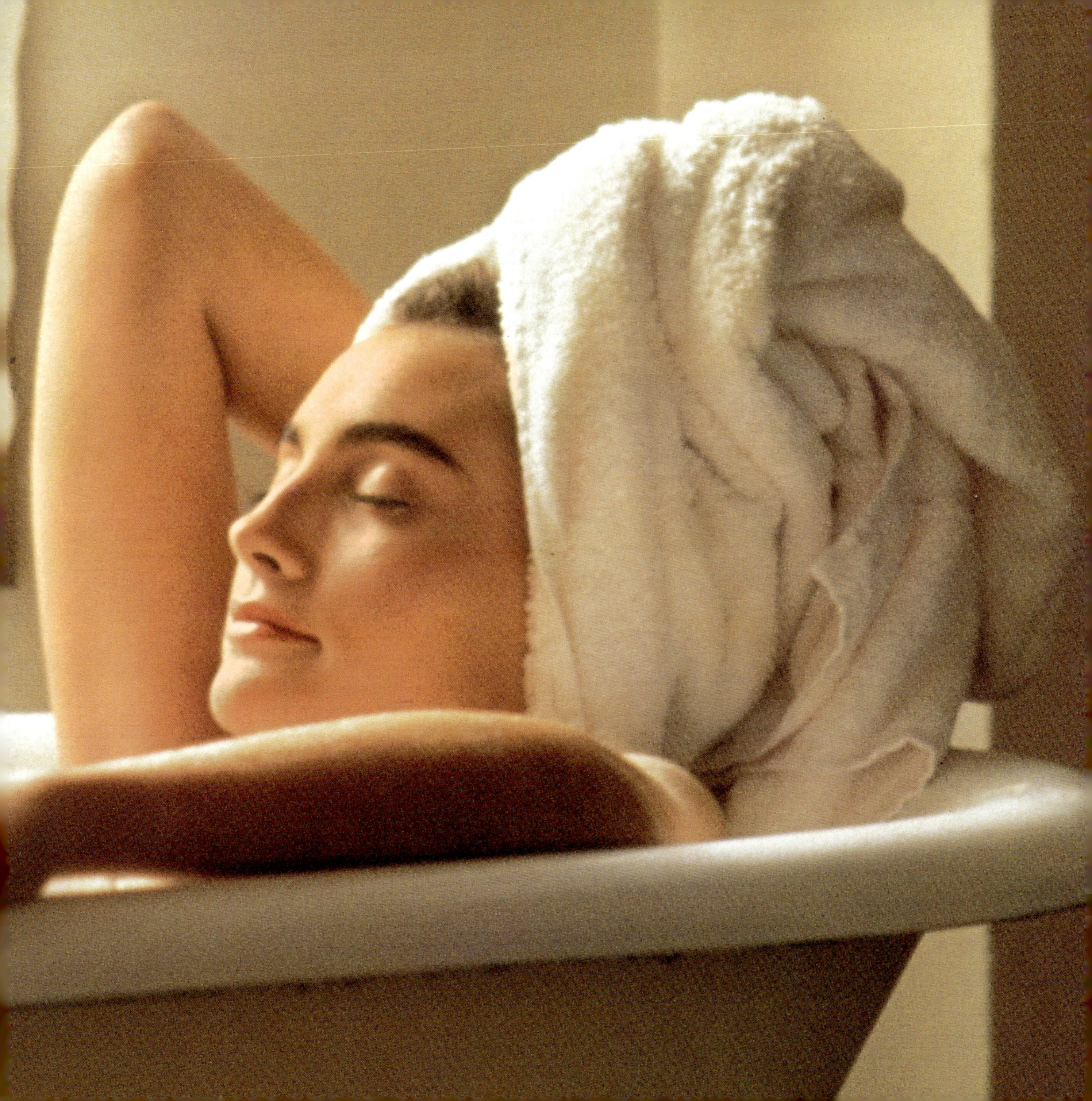

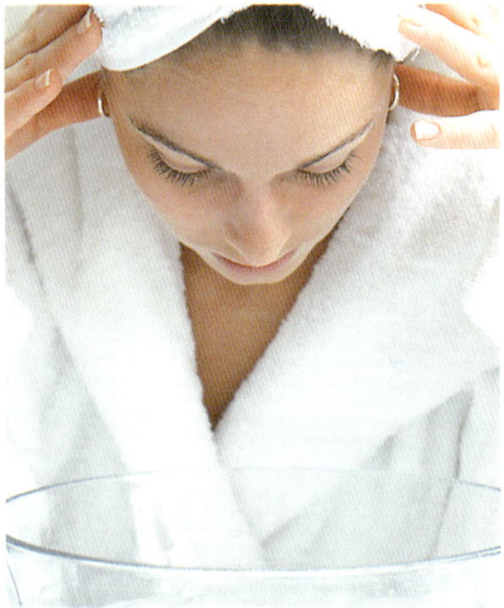

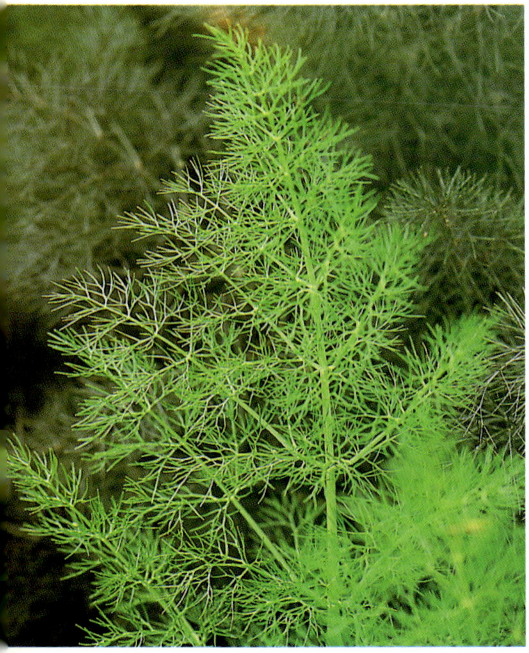

purifying

Plants have been used for thousands of years to cleanse and purify and those with a fresh "medicinal" smell are useful if you need to give your body a detox or simply want to keep the surrounding air clean and germ-free.

Two of the most important purifying plants, tea tree and eucalyptus, originate in Australia. Tea tree, which has been long known to the Australian Aborigines, has powerful antiseptic, antifungal and antibacterial properties. Its sharp, pungent and camphorous aroma is ideal for use in a vaporizer to kill airborne germs.

The piercingly fresh, menthol vapour of eucalyptus is also perfectly suited for use as a cleanser, and is effective as both a preventative and a remedy. Its smell has a head-clearing and cooling effect and can bring down a fever. If your sinuses are blocked it can be a powerful antidote. Try taking a sauna, add three to four drops to the bucket of water, mix well and pour over the hot coals. The aromatic steam will have an instant effect.

Juniper has a long history of medical use. Until recently, sprigs of juniper, together with rosemary, were burnt in French hospitals to cleanse and purify the air, releasing a distinctive fresh and woody aroma. Juniper also has a strong, detoxifying effect on the body and combines well with fennel, another disinfectant and purifier, which has a fresh, aniseed-like smell. For treating cellulite, both juniper and fennel are very helpful: add a few drops each of fennel and juniper essential oil to a massage base oil and rub on to the affected areas daily.

left Graceful feathery fennel has been used since Roman times for both culinary and medicinal purposes. The Roman historian Pliny listed it as a remedy for no fewer than 22 complaints.

top and opposite Clear blocked sinuses with a revitalizing burst of the fresh, menthol smell from plants such as eucalyptus and tea tree.

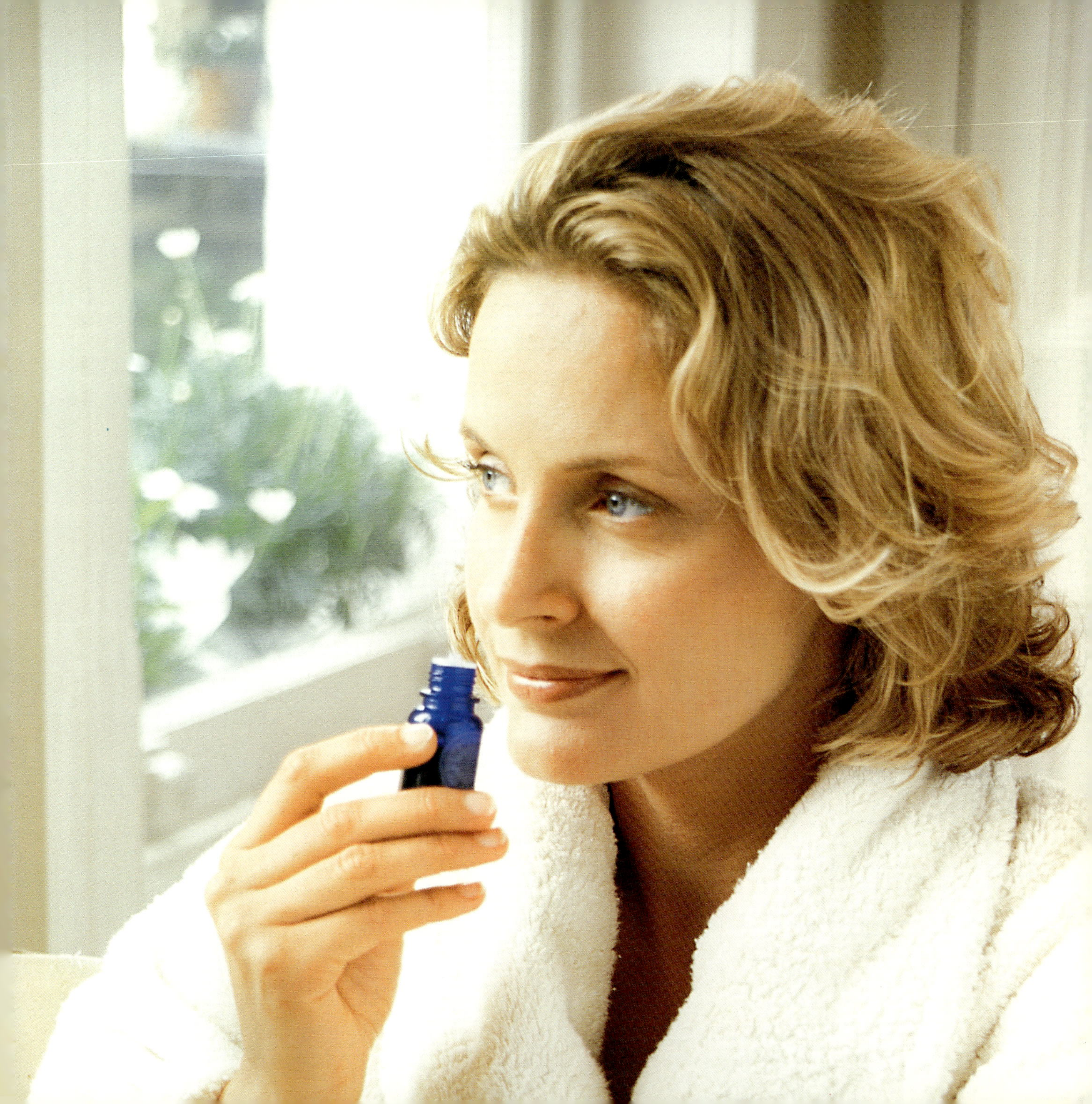

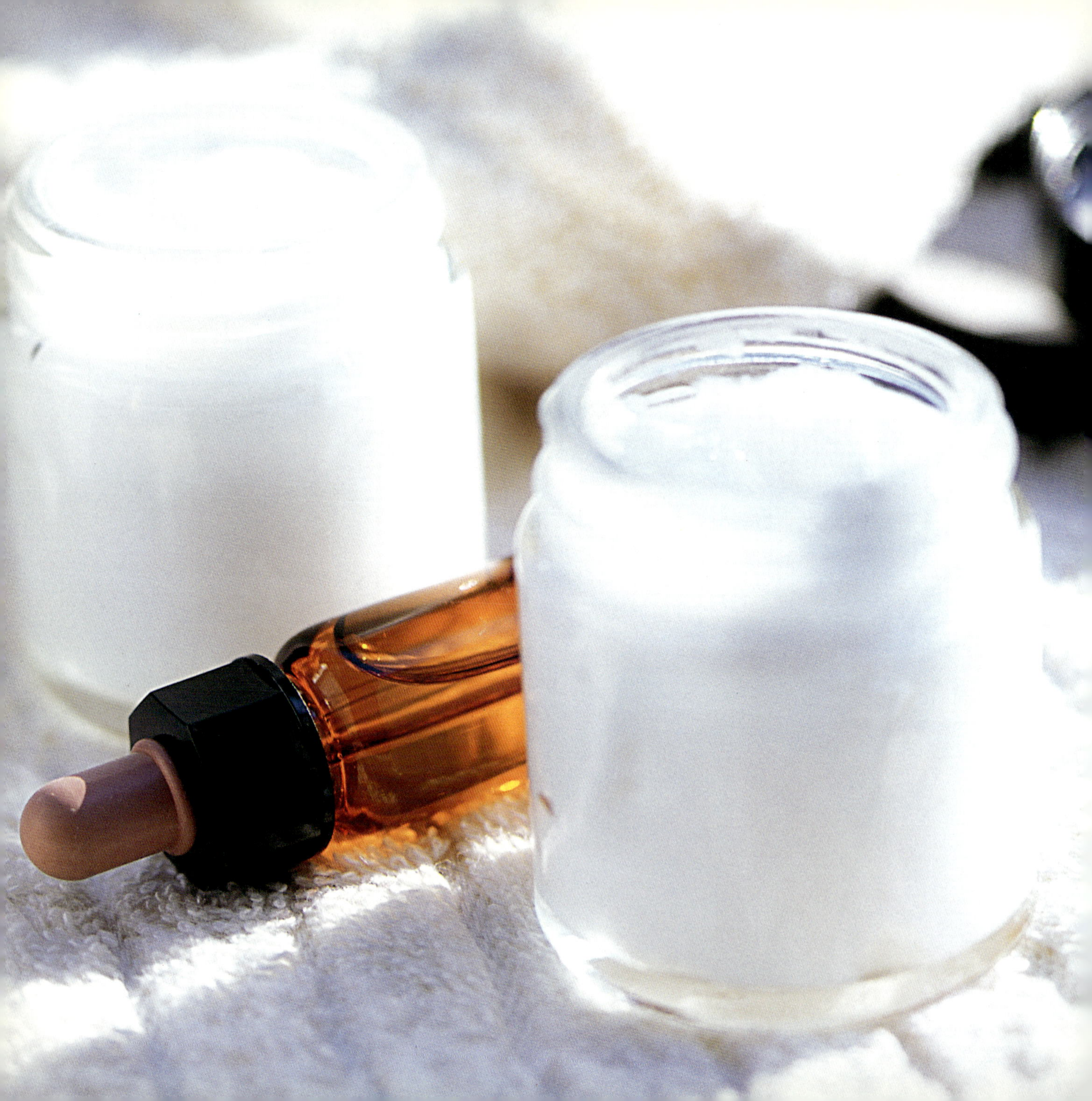

regenerating

Even if there is no magical potion we can take to keep us forever young, there are certain plants that stimulate the growth of healthy new cells in the human body, most notably lavender and neroli.

The healing properties of lavender, known to the ancients for thousands of years, were rediscovered in the 20th century when a French chemist, René-Maurice Gattefossé, accidentally burnt his arm. He plunged his arm into a jar of lavender oil, and was astonished at how quickly his wound healed, with very little scarring. Lavender is not only a powerful skin rejuvenator, it also helps normalize both dry and greasy skins and can be used for treating difficult skin conditions, such as acne: try adding a few drops to an unperfumed body lotion or face cream.

Weak, brittle or damaged nails can also benefit from lavender's strengthening properties. To encourage strong, healthy nails, you have to care for the cuticle as well as the nail as this is where nail growth begins: each evening, rub a few drops of lavender oil into the cuticles. After two or three months you should see some improvement as the treated nail grows through.

The delicate oil of neroli is widely used in commercially made perfume and skincare products and is particularly beneficial for dry or sensitive skin. It helps eliminate dead skin cells, improves the skin's elasticity, and is useful for all kinds of skin problems, including thread veins and stretch marks.

Regular use of both lavender and neroli oils in baths and in massage can help to maintain cellular reproduction at the levels that occur naturally in young people. Try experimenting with these oils on a daily basis, by adding a few drops to face creams, body lotions and/or bath oils.

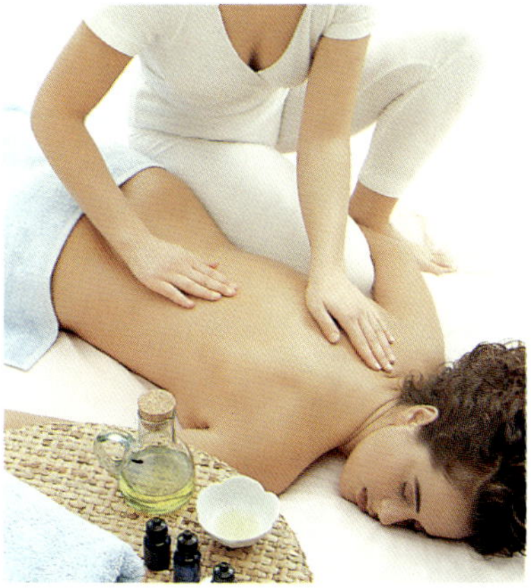

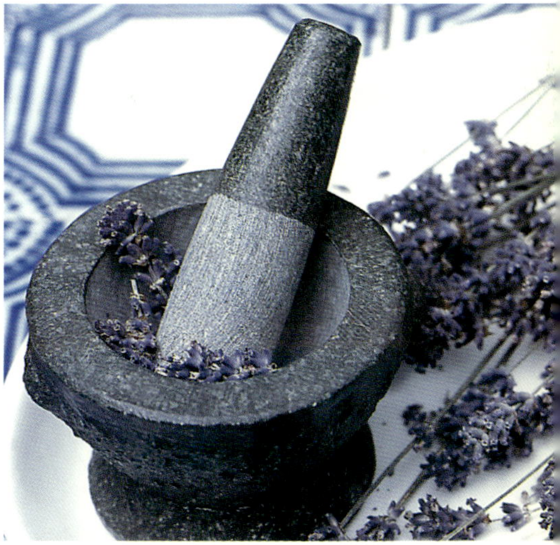

opposite Use essential oils in the daily care of your skin to keep it supple and youthful.
top and above Lavender has long been valued for its healing qualities, as well as its unmistakable perfume, and is particularly beneficial in massage.

pampering treats

Looking after our skin is a chance for pampering and rejuvenating, and there is nothing like using your own home-made products to create a real sense of wellbeing.

nourishing night cream

As we get older, our skin becomes drier and in need of regular care. Jasmine and rose oils help to rehydrate the skin, while frankincense helps reduce wrinkles and restore tone to slack muscles.

you will need:
50g/2oz jar of unperfumed base cream
with a close-fitting lid
3 drops of rose essential oil
2 drops of frankincense essential oil
1 drop of jasmine essential oil

Add the oils to the cream, and mix well together. Apply a little of the cream just before going to bed.

lavender and olive oil soap

Use a good quality pure olive-oil soap for this lovely home-made soap. Enrich it with other oils and scent it with lavender for a gently rejuvenating cleanser.

you will need:
175g/6oz good quality olive-oil soap
25ml/1fl oz coconut oil
25ml/1fl oz almond oil
30ml/2 tbsp ground almonds
10 drops of lavender essential oil

Grate the soap and place in a double boiler. Leave the soap to soften over a low heat. When soft, add all the other ingredients. Stir well, until all the ingredients are evenly mixed and begin to hold together. Press the mixture into oiled moulds and leave to set overnight. Unmould and decorate by pressing the top of each block of soap into a shallow tray of lavender buds.

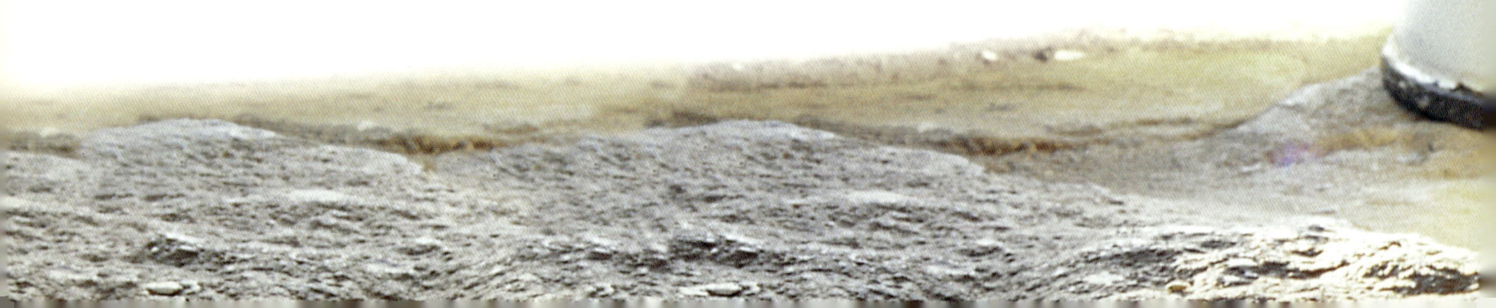

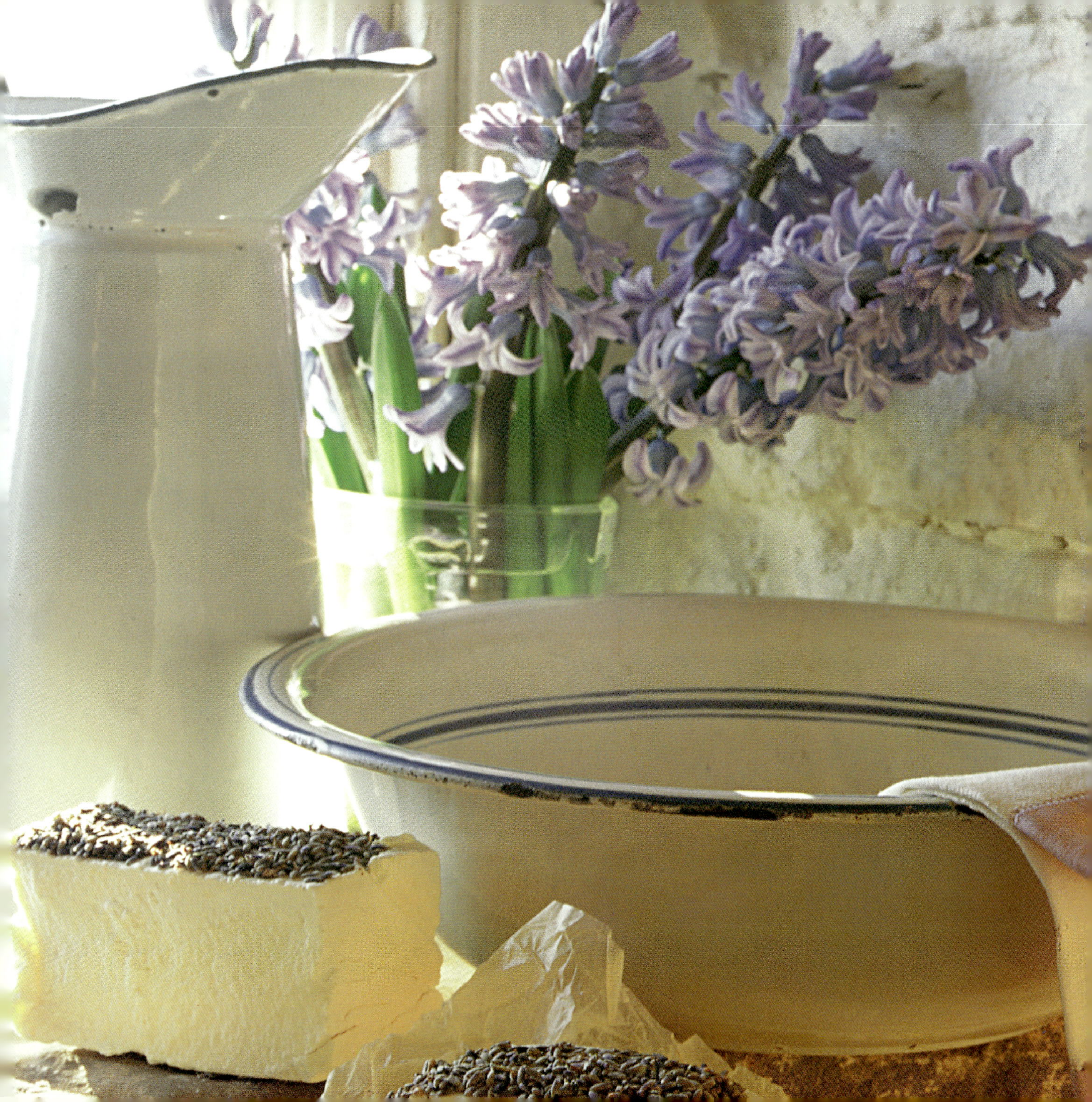

warm and comforting

In winter, there is nothing quite like rich, pungent and spicy aromas to bring warmth and vitality into our homes and to create a mellow and inviting ambience. Packed into the bark, roots, seeds, flowers and even the stamens of some plants is an explosion of spicy fragrance and flavour that has been used in cooking since ancient times, as well as for scenting and healing.

The warm, spicy smell of nutmeg has a soft and evocative effect and is said to stimulate dreams, while the penetratingly hot and sweet fragrance of cloves aids the recollection of long-forgotten memories. If you enjoy sitting at the fireside and reminiscing with friends, either of these aromas will help create the right mood.

Cinnamon is also useful for strengthening the immune system and protecting against colds and flu. This exotic spice has a hot, sharp and slightly sweet aroma. It helps to relieve aches and chills felt in the early stages of a cold, and is a good antidote for stomach upsets. Highly prized for its culinary and medicinal uses, cinnamon is among the oldest and most sought-after spices known: at one time, it was more valuable than gold.

Both cinnamon and cloves blend well with orange to make a wonderful winter fragrance. For Christmas parties, make an aromatic mulled wine punch, using red wine and a little added sugar with slices of orange, some cinnamon sticks and a few clove buds.

When the nights draw in, rich, pungent, spicy aromas surround us with warmth and vitality, and create a mellow and inviting ambience in our homes.

On a practical level, cloves are a powerful antiseptic and give good protection against winter illnesses. The oil is valued for its ability to help clear chesty coughs and blocked sinuses. To ward off infections, vaporize a few drops in a burner.

top left Placing a hot dish on this clove-filled cushion releases the tantalizing scent of the spice.
bottom left Cloves are an antiseptic and can have a mild anaesthetic effect; traditionally the oil was used to relieve toothache.

top right Elegant and richly coloured quills of cinnamon are used in cooking around the world.
bottom right For a traditional fragrant pomander, stud an orange with cloves, then toss in orris root and ground cinnamon and hang.

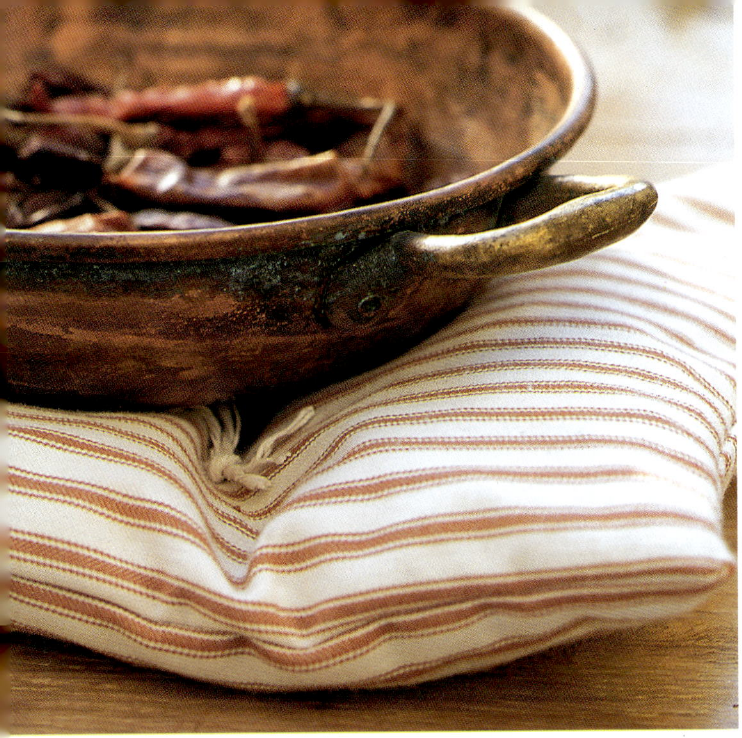
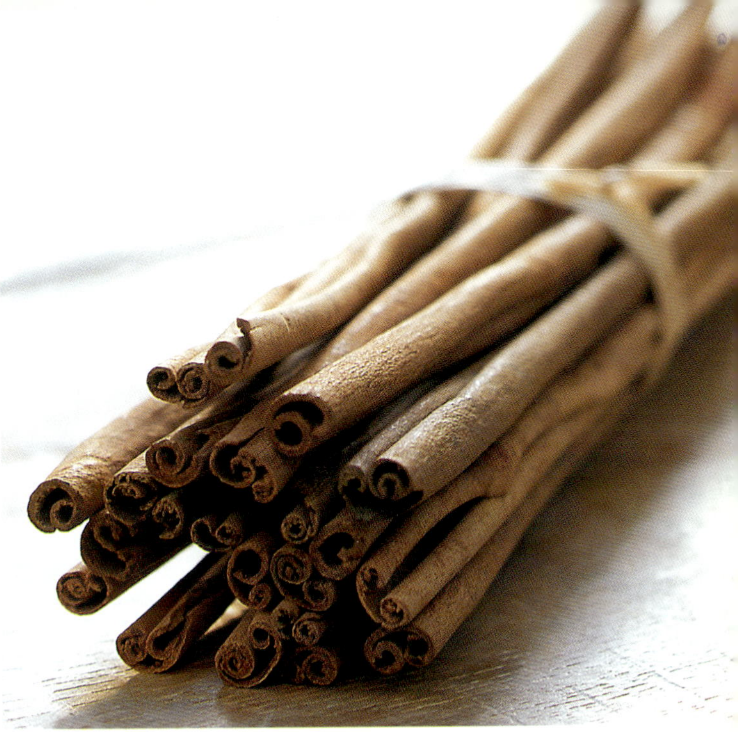
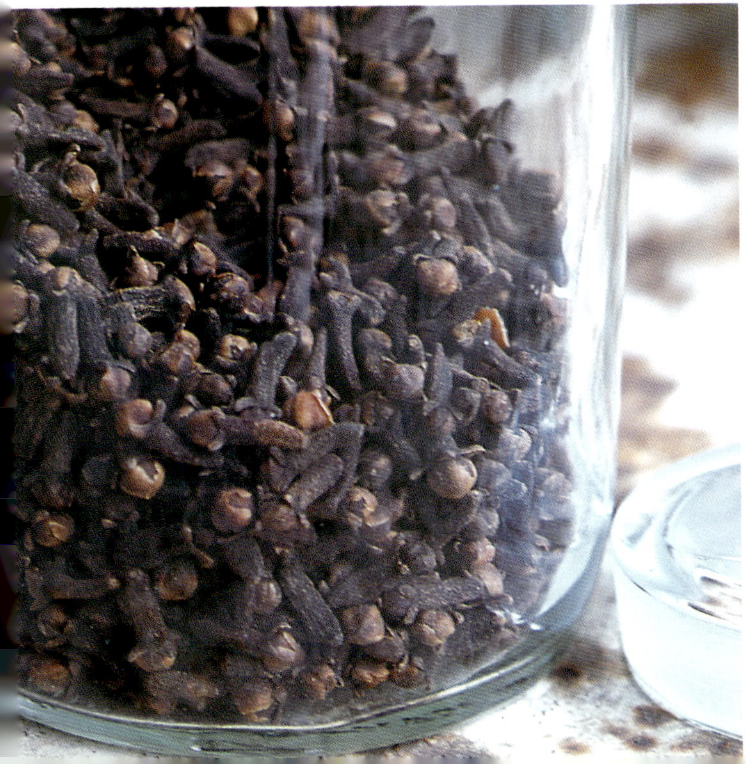
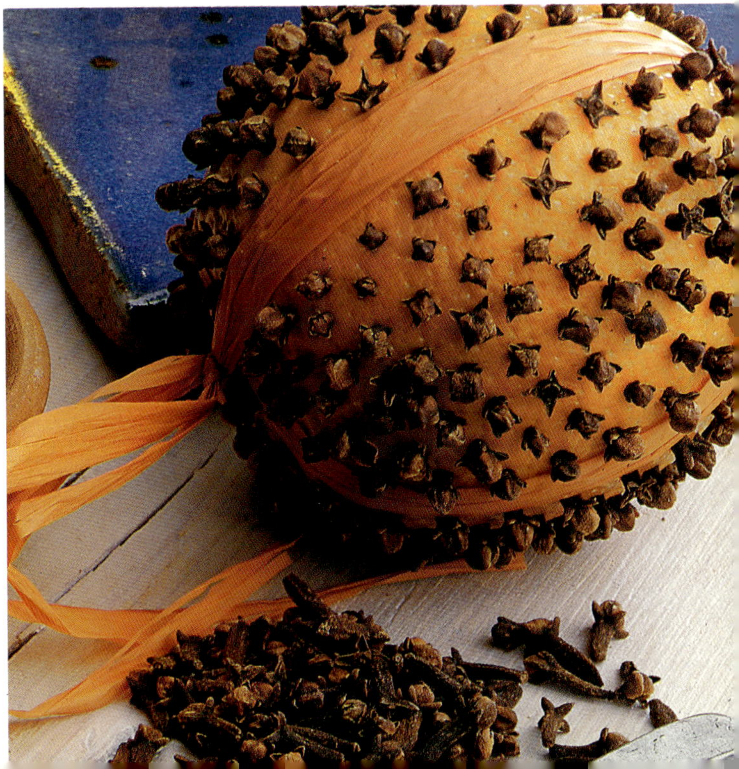

sensual and seductive

We all need a little pampering every now and then, and some scents and flowers seem almost synonymous with luxury, whether in the form of a simple posy of fresh flowers or as fabulously evocative essential oils used in a warm bath. In particular, certain fragrances, such as rose, jasmine, neroli and ylang ylang, are well-known aphrodisiacs, and there are a variety of ways they can be used to bring a little romance into your daily life.

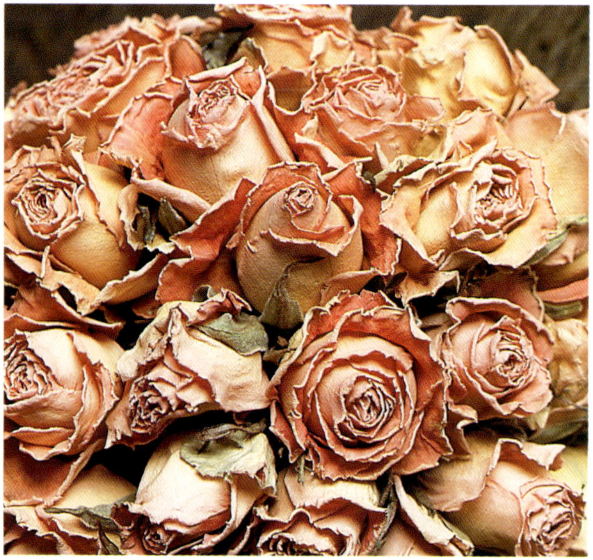

above This glorious rose pomander is a modern adaption of the traditional variety, and is scented with neroli and rose essential oils.

The exquisitely scented rose is the classic symbol of romance and seduction, and is associated with Aphrodite, the Greek goddess of love, beauty and fertility. Cleopatra knew of its powers and it is said that Mark Antony had to wade knee-deep through red rose petals to reach her bed. Thankfully, there are many other, less extravagant, ways to experience the powers of rose: in pot pourri or dried flowers, in perfume and in eau de Colognes. To make an undeniably sensuous bath oil, mix rose essential oil with that of sandalwood; the scent will linger on your skin long after the bath.

If rose is regarded as the Queen of Flowers, then jasmine is considered King. Although the white flowers are delicately shaped, their long-lasting fragrance is of a more masculine nature: rich, musky and earthy. Like rose, jasmine is a remedy for sexual frigidity and impotence, helping to relax and calm the body – use a little of the oil in the bath or in massage.

The richly scented yellow blooms of ylang ylang have an exotic and voluptuous, sweet and heady aroma. The term ylang ylang means "flower of flowers" in the Malay language, and the blooms are used by native women in Indonesia to perfume their hair, and are spread on the beds of newly-weds to calm wedding-night nerves. Renowned for their ability to relax and seduce, they help slow down an over rapid breathing rate and heartbeat.

Of a gentler nature, neroli is one of the finest floral essences and is often used in eau de Cologne. It comes from the bitter orange tree whose flowers are used in bridal bouquets and garlands to symbolize innocence and to secure love. The simple, sweet fragrance of neroli brings happiness and nourishment to the soul.

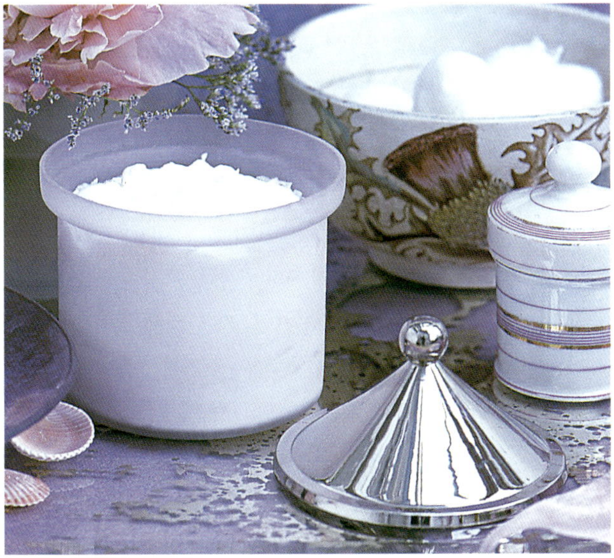

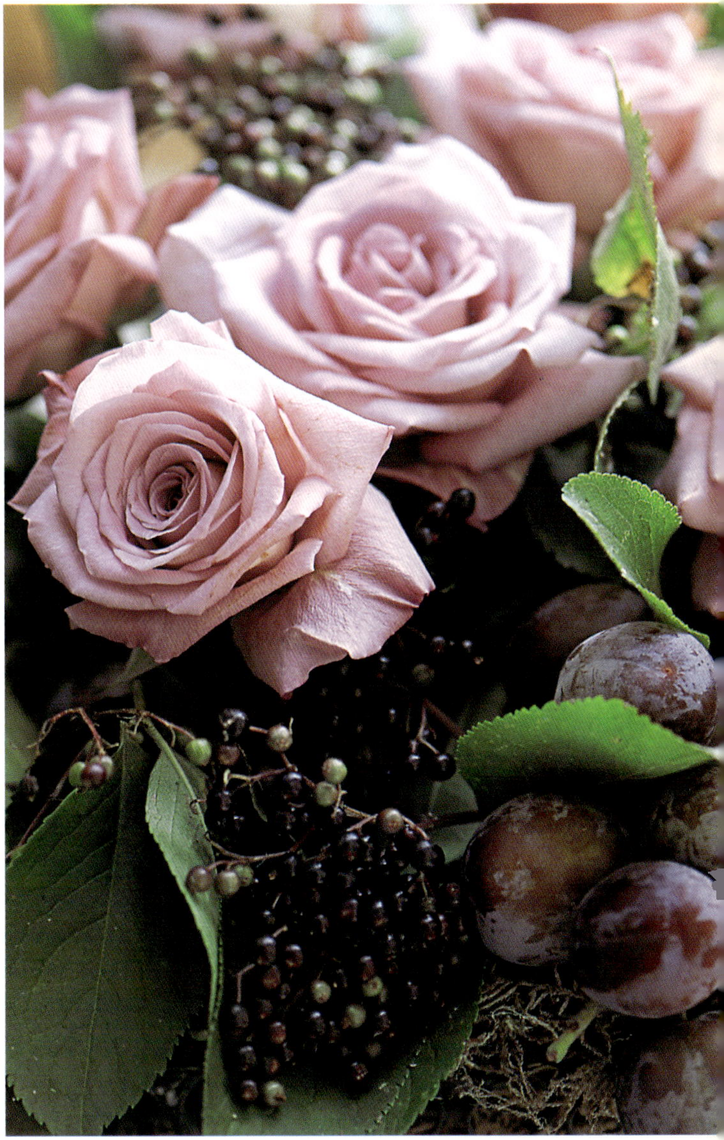

above and right Certain flowers, such as the rose, seem to symbolize luxury and are delightful in many forms, from lotions to floral displays.

the sensual sanctuary

We all know that it is important to occasionally indulge ourselves, and our partners, but how often do we actually do so? Creating a sensual haven – even if just for an hour or two – is one of the best ways of doing this.

The bedroom and bathroom are two places where it is fairly easy to create the right atmosphere. Dim the lights, play appropriate music, and select scents to suit your mood. Use creams, lotions, floral waters or perfumes to spoil yourself with, and enjoy a relaxing, luxurious bath or a sensual massage.

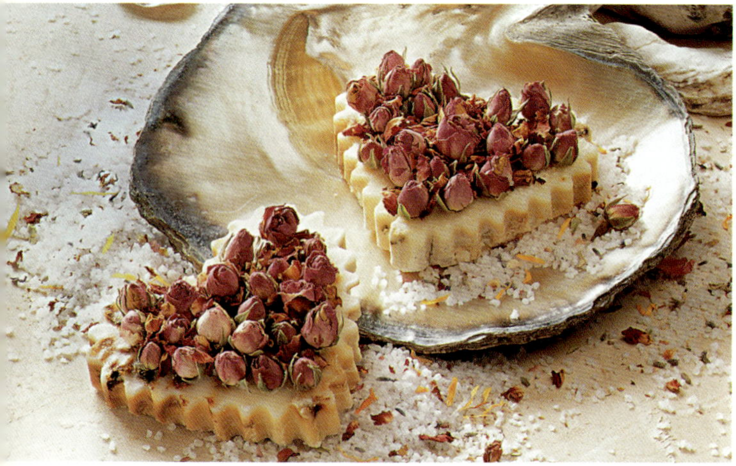

above and opposite Whether alone, or with another, use scented rose soap, candles and chilled wine to add a touch of decadence to bathing.

rose and sandalwood bath oil

Use this luxurious oil sparingly; a little will go a long way. The warm, spicy fragrance will linger on your skin after your bath.

you will need:

100ml/3½fl oz almond oil

20ml/4 tsp wheatgerm oil

15 drops of rose essential oil

10 drops of sandalwood essential oil

seductive massage mix

There is nothing like giving and receiving a massage to relax tension and create intimacy.

you will need:

105ml/7 tbsp grapeseed oil

5ml/1 tsp wheatgerm oil

5 drops of rose essential oil

3 drops of ylang ylang essential oil

2 drops of jasmine essential oil

For both blends, combine the ingredients and store in a dark-coloured screw-top bottle. Use as required.

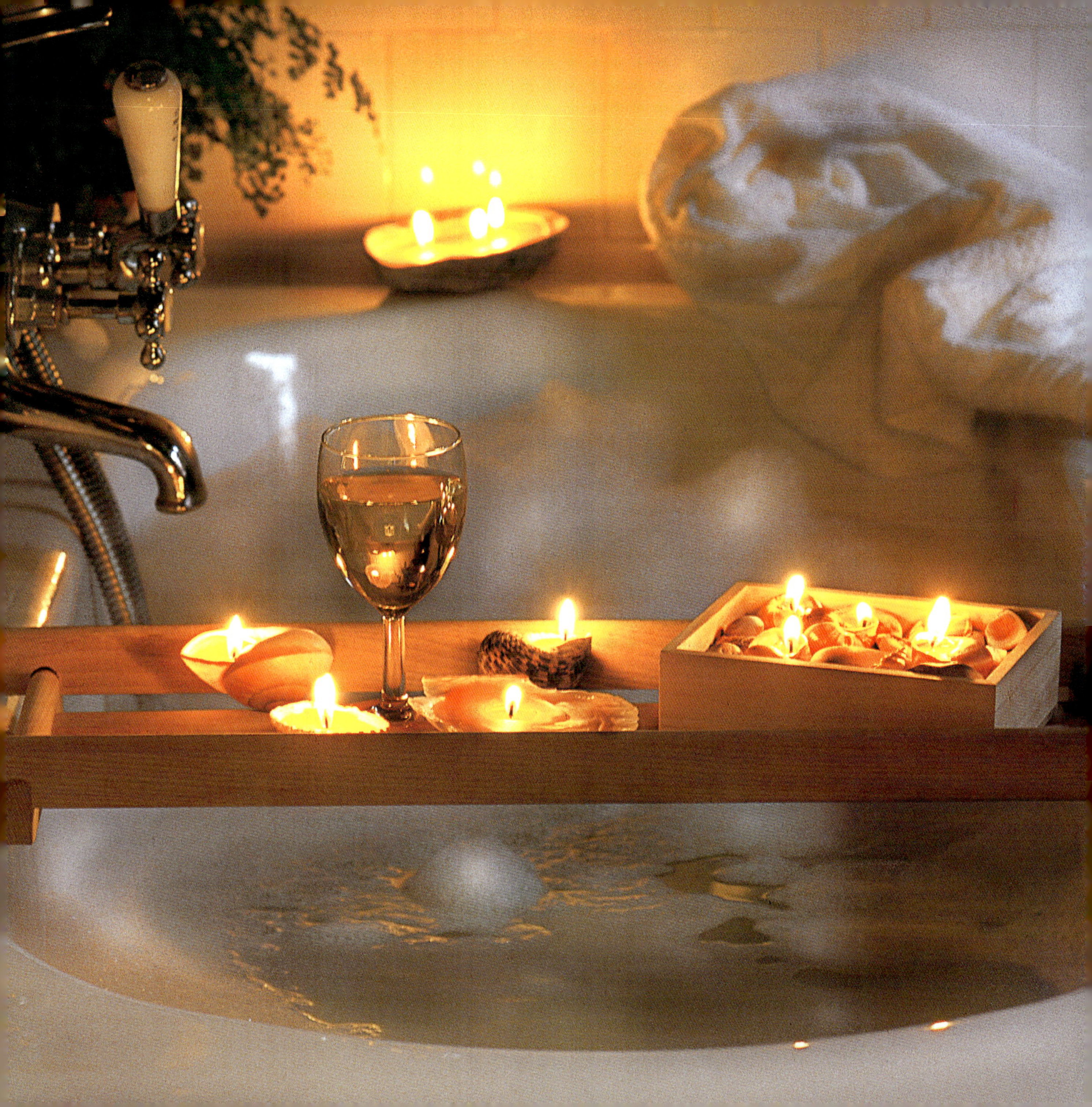

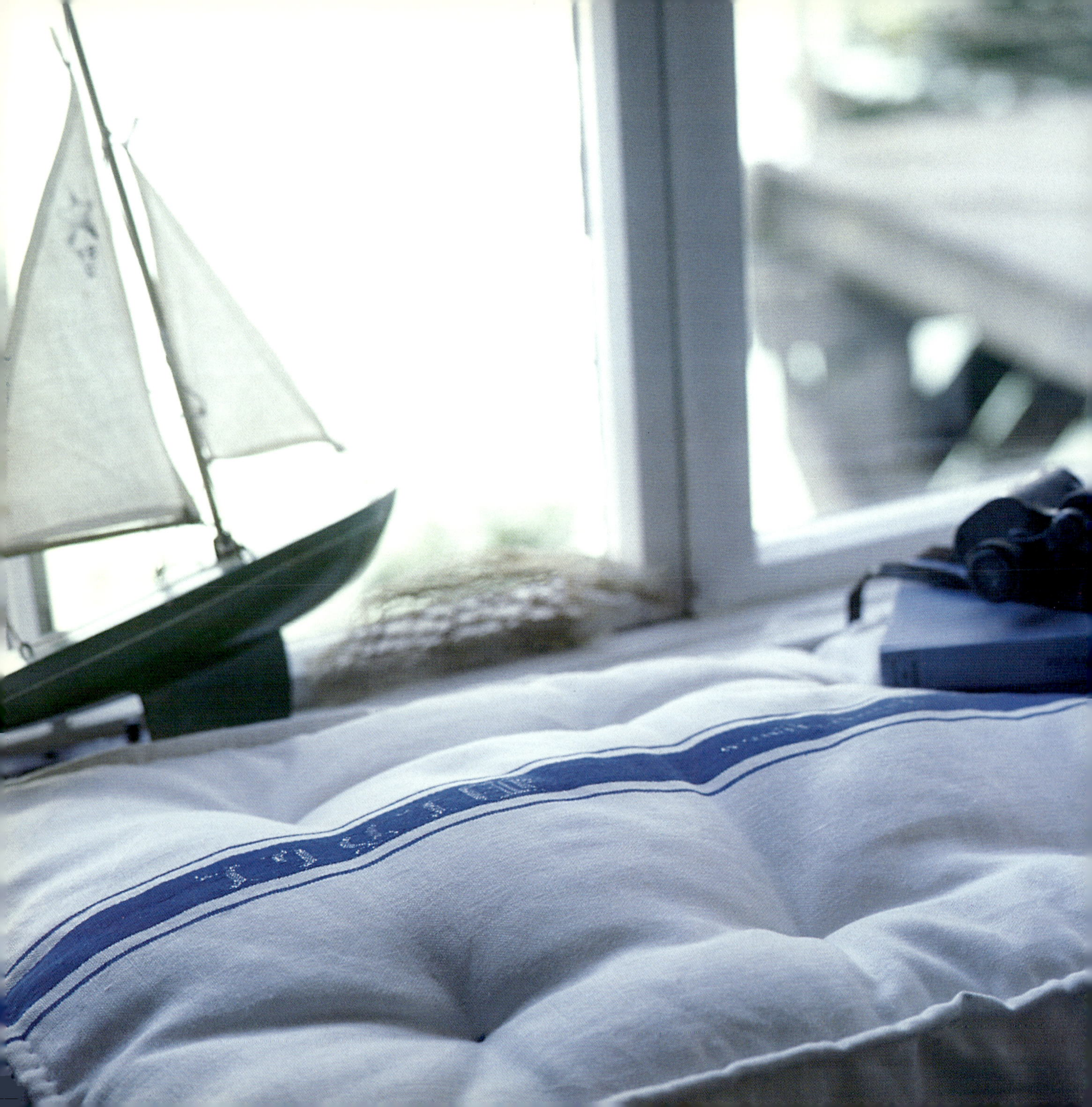

relaxing

Modern life is busy and stressful: make time to sit or rest quietly for a few moments each day, close your eyes, breathe slowly and let your mind go. To further help you, experiment with fragrances such as myrrh, frankincense and sandalwood, whose very names conjure up mysterious and exotic otherworlds that are far from the everyday.

The ancient Egyptians believed that the smoky and mysterious aroma of myrrh was particularly pleasing to the gods. Like frankincense, myrrh heightens an awareness of higher levels of consciousness. Use when you are agitated: its cooling fragrance will help put everyday worries into perspective.

Valued as highly as gold, frankincense was one of the gifts of the Kings to Jesus. The vapour is balsamic and spicy, with a warming and calming effect. Frankincense deepens and slows the breath, thus helping the mind and body to relax and producing a heightened awareness of the spiritual realm.

Sandalwood is probably the oldest known perfume in history, with more than 4,000 years of recorded use. Prized in India, the wood was used to build temples, carved into icons, and burned as incense. This musky, exotic aroma facilitates meditation and is favoured by yogis to encourage a contemplative state.

All three of these perfumes can be used separately or in combination. Try burning them as incense, or vaporize the oils in a burner.

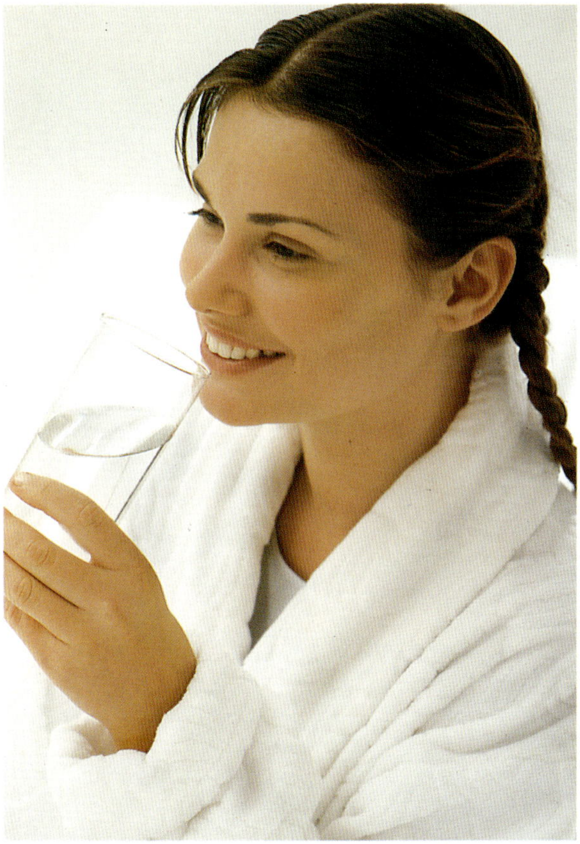

opposite and above Use scents to conjure up thoughts of holidays and far-away places. Vaporize a few drops of frankincense oil combined with lavender oil to create a tranquil and relaxing atmosphere – one that is just right for dreaming.

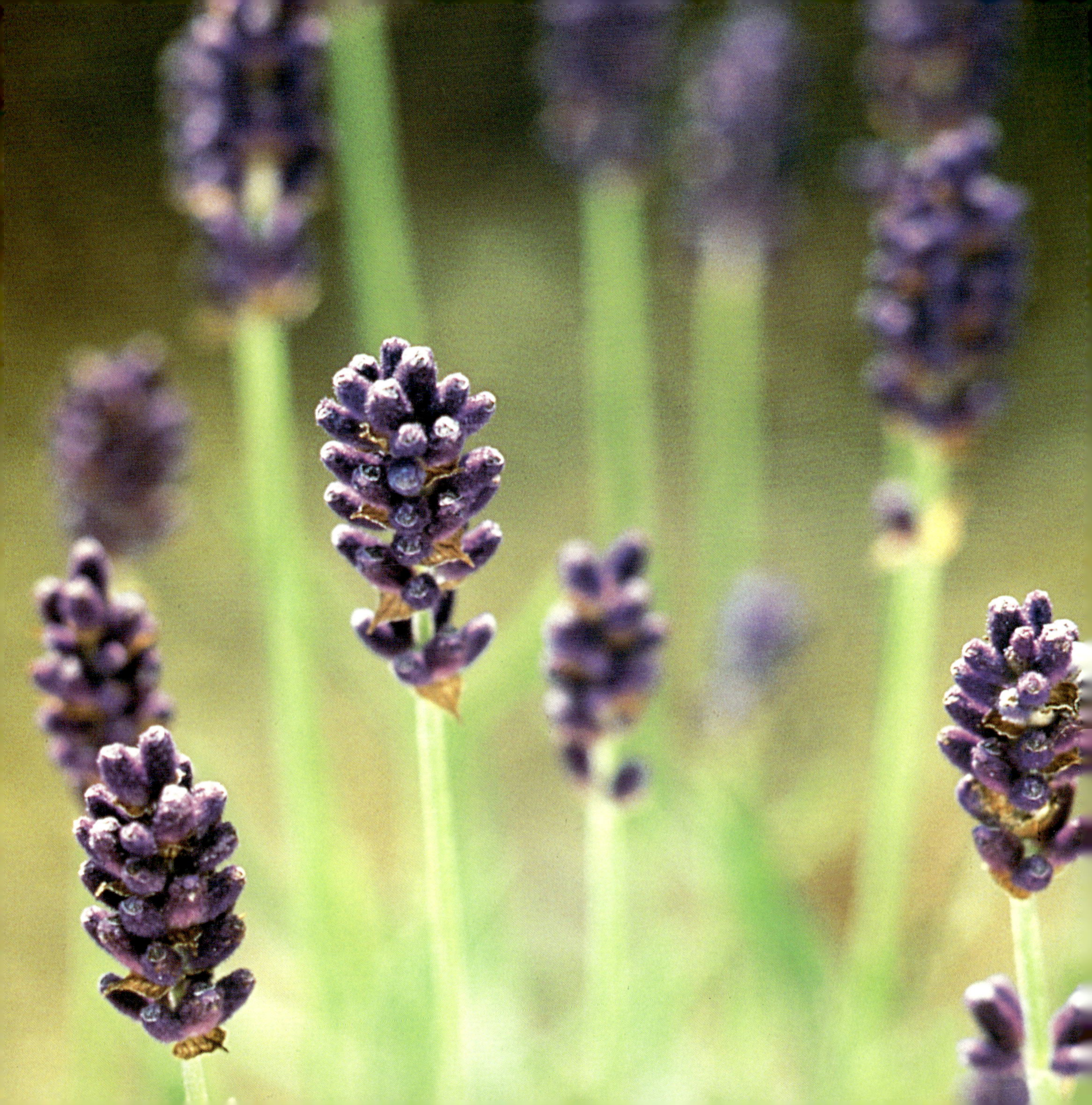

a guide to scents

When fragrance is used for pleasure alone, the choice is usually based on an individual's preference for the aroma. When used to maintain or improve health, however, the properties and effects of a scent are a crucial part of the choice. This section discusses the most common ways of using scents at home, as well as providing a handy checklist of the different properties of the aromas included in this book. Scents are powerful, concentrated substances – it is important to understand how they work, so that they can be used safely and effectively, and if in doubt seek medical advice. Treat them with care and respect and allow them to treat you.

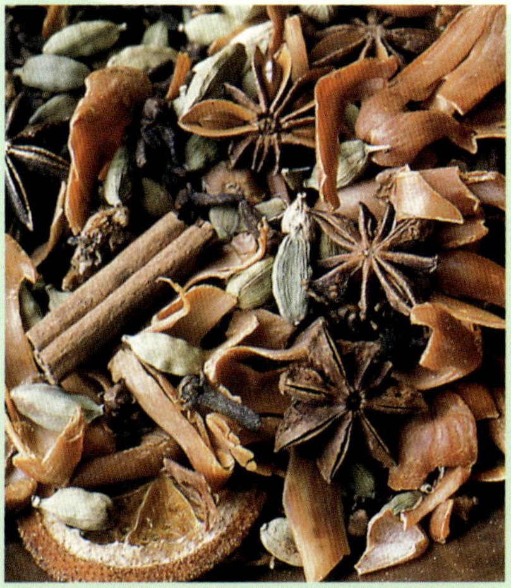

using scents

We can benefit from many parts of the scented plant – fresh and/or dried plant constituents such as petals, leaves, bark and seeds, as well as the distilled essential oil. There are also many ways we can use these products, such as in massage and baths, inhalation, food and drink, and in the air around us.

Before embarking on any treatment using essential oils, it is important to know a little bit about how they work in order to use them safely. The two primary ways of using oils at home are by inhalation or by application to the skin in a carrier oil. When we breathe in scents, some oil molecules travel to the lungs to be absorbed into the blood. Other molecules go directly to the brain, which then releases neurochemicals that act on the person. When scented products are applied to the body, the chemical compounds from the plant extract are absorbed by the skin into the bloodstream and lymphatic system, from where they can travel to any part of the body. Essential oils are concentrated substances, and are always diluted in a carrier base oil before being used on the body. Good quality oils, such as almond, wheatgerm, jojoba and avocado, make excellent carriers. Alternatively, essential oils can be added to water and used for bathing, misting on to the skin or vaporizing.

Always handle essential oils with care and consideration – they are highly powerful, medicinal substances. If in any doubt, seek an expert medical opinion before using them.

- Use only good quality, unadulterated essential oils.
- Store essential oils, scents and perfumes away from the light in a fairly cool position.
- Essential oils are highly concentrated substances, and should not be taken internally nor applied directly to the skin.
- Always use in diluted form, mixed with a suitable carrier base of vegetable oil or added to bath water, for example. Carry out a patch test on a small area of skin if using an oil for the first time.
- Certain essential oils should be avoided completely during pregnancy: seek professional guidance if unsure.
- Essential oils should not be used for children under 2 years of age.
- Avoid getting undiluted plant essences in the eyes, as this can cause permanent damage.
- Certain essential oils, particularly the citrus ones, should not be used for two hours before exposure to sunlight or a sunbed.

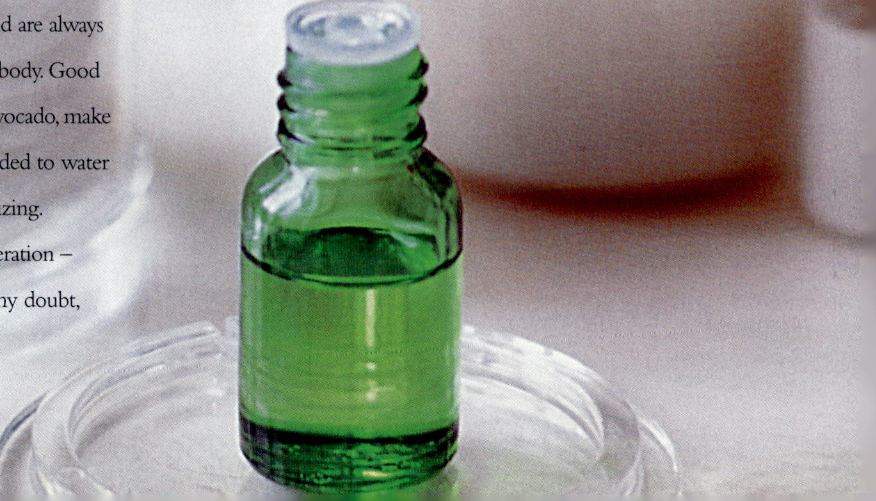

scenting the body

The best way to use a scent on the body is to "layer" it, by using a variety of scented products. So a bath oil, soap, dusting powder, body lotion and eau de toilette will each add a layer of fragrance, some of which will evaporate into the air, while the rest will be absorbed by the skin to pleasantly linger over many hours. Just make sure that your scents harmonize with one another and don't compete for attention.

massage There is no better way to pamper your body. An essential oil blended with almond or wheatgerm oil makes a perfect massage oil. Blend in the proportion of 2–3 drops of essential oil to 15ml/1 tbsp carrier oil.

bathtime A scented bath is one of life's luxuries. Choose two or three essential oils and use 8–10 drops altogether. Add the oils to a warm bath and swish the water thoroughly to disperse them. Alternatively, mix the drops of oil beforehand in a little almond oil, or a little milk, and add to the bath. Lower the water temperature for a more stimulating soak.

skincare After a bath or shower, nourish your skin with scented creams and lotions. Use an unperfumed cream and add 3–4 drops of essential oil to 30ml/2 tbsp cream. For a lotion with a thinner consistency, add jojoba or avocado oil to the mix.

footbath If you suffer from swollen feet and tired, aching legs, a footbath is a real treat. Add 6–8 drops of essential oil to a bowl of warm water and soak your feet for 10 minutes.

muscle rub To warm up the body before an exercise workout, choose invigorating or stimulating fragrances: add 1 drop of essential oil to 5ml/1 tsp carrier oil. For aching muscles, choose fragrances that have a relaxing effect.

compresses Use cool compresses for acute pain and injury, and warm ones to alleviate swelling and to reduce inflammation. Mix 3–5 drops of essential oil in a bowl of hot or cold water and soak a piece of soft cotton until the oils are absorbed. Apply the soaked pad to the affected area. Compresses are useful for treating insect bites, painful joints, stomach pains and headache.

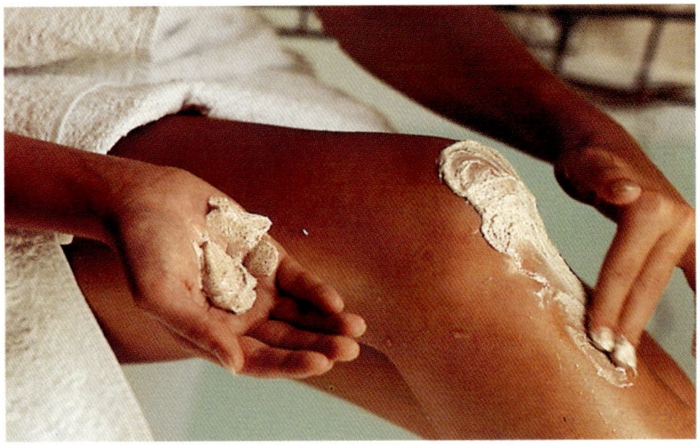

above Mix scented creams or lotions with a carrier base oil to make them go further.

using inhalations

The fastest way to benefit from a fragrance is by inhalation: nerve pathways lead from the lining of the nose to the part of the brain that deals with memory and emotions.

tissue inhalation Sprinkle a few drops of essential oil on a tissue, keep it with you and sniff throughout the day. This is a particularly good way to simply and easily combat stress or work pressures in the office.

steam inhalation These are great for clearing blocked sinuses. Add 5 drops of essential oil to a bowl of steaming water. Carefully lean over the bowl, cover your head and the bowl with a towel to make a tent and breathe in deeply.

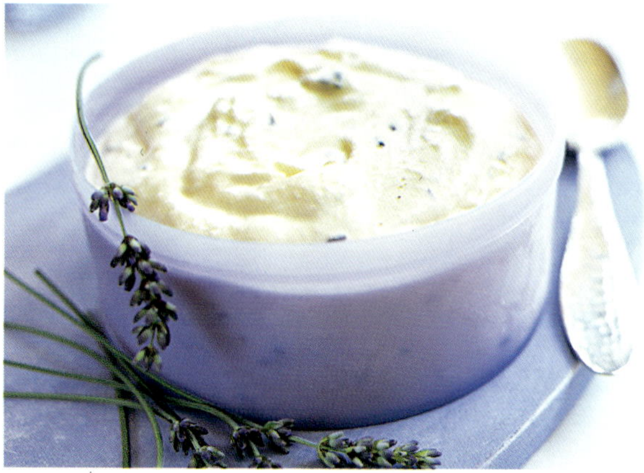

above Ice-cream scented with lavender makes a pretty and gently aromatic dish.

sauna During winter, antiviral essential oils, such as eucalyptus and pine, work well in the sauna. Mix 3–4 drops of oil in the water bucket and splash on to the hot coals.

nourishing the body

Fragrant spices and herbs – even edible flowers – can add considerably to our enjoyment of food and drink and can be highly beneficial. It is not advisable to take essential oils internally without medical supervision.

food and drink Use aromatic spices to pep up your cooking, eat fragrant herbs in salads and sauces, and make healthy herbal, fruit and spice drinks. Spiced and herbal oils and vinegars also make wonderful gifts.

infusions Herbal teas or *tisanes* are made by boiling in water the soft leaves, stems or flowers of a plant, and then straining off the liquid. Chamomile flowers combined with mint leaves makes a refreshing summer drink.

decoctions For a stronger, spicy brew, use the bark and roots of a plant. Use 25g/1oz whole spices to 900ml/ 1½ pints/3¾ cups water. Boil until the liquid is reduced to 600ml/1 pint/2½ cups, then strain, discarding the spices.

scenting your home

A pleasant smell is usually the first thing you notice when you enter a room, and it can strongly affect your mood. Use aromas not only to feel good but also to purify the air.

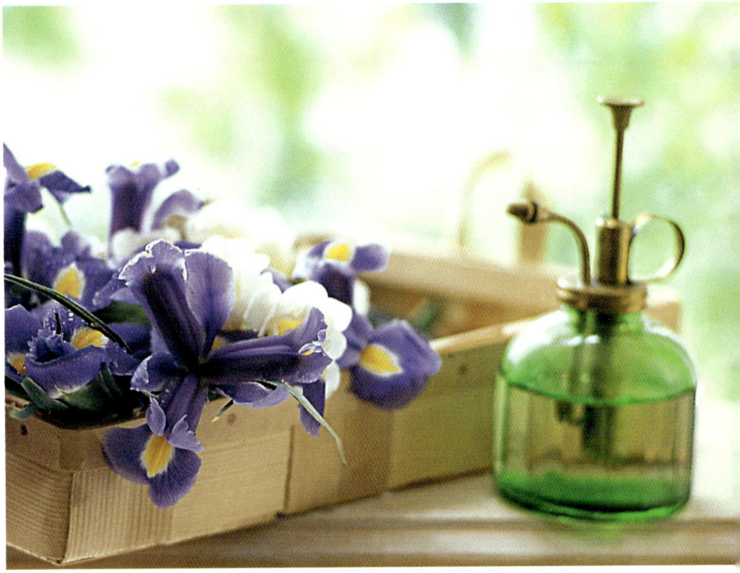

above Use your favourite scents in a misting bottle, mixed with a little water, to freshen up the air around the house.

spritzer To freshen up a stale atmosphere, blend 10 drops of essential oil, such as rose, with 105ml/7 tbsp water and mix well, then add to a misting bottle. Spray into the air as needed.

potpourri The natural fragrance of potpourri is perfect for subtle, long-term room scenting. Use a mixture of dried leaves, twigs, petals and buds and dried fruit and nuts. Add a few drops of essential oil and use a fixative (powdered orris root is the best) to preserve the scent.

pomanders These perfumed balls were at one time carried as protection against infection. Today, citrus pomanders are used mainly as festive decorations, but they are also effective in warding off insects. Stud oranges, lemons or kumquats with cloves and toss in ground cinnamon and orris root. Leave to dry out for a few weeks then hang.

firesticks Dried herbs, roots, seeds and plant constituents will perfume a room if put on an open fire when the flames are low. Try pine cones, lavender bundles, or sage.

scented linen For old-fashioned luxury, scent linen with the delicate fragrance of flowers and plants. Make tiny cushions and fill with dried lavender heads, or sprinkle oils of lemon grass, cedarwood and rosewood on to drawer liners.

vaporizers These come in many forms, but essentially consist of a shallow bowl standing over a small chamber containing a night-light. Fill the bowl with warm water, add 2–3 drops of essential oil and light the night-light. As the water is heated the oil vaporizes its perfume.

summertime scents

Chamomile

botanical name *Anthemis nobilis*

family *Asteraceae*

Roman chamomile is native to the British Isles and is a small perennial with feathery leaves and daisy-like flowers. The essential oil has a fragrance resembling over-ripe apples. Its action is gentle, soothing and calming, making it suitable for babies. Chamomile flowers are widely drunk in teas.

properties analgesic, anti-anaemic, antiseptic, anti-inflammatory, antineuralgic, antispasmodic, calming and sedative, digestive, diuretic

uses *body* useful for rheumatic inflammation, indigestion, headaches, menstrual problems *mind* can alleviate hysteria, nervous afflictions, fear, insomnia *spirit* brings patience and peace, helps to reinstate a feeling of comfort and belonging

cautions avoid using the essential oil during the first three months of pregnancy

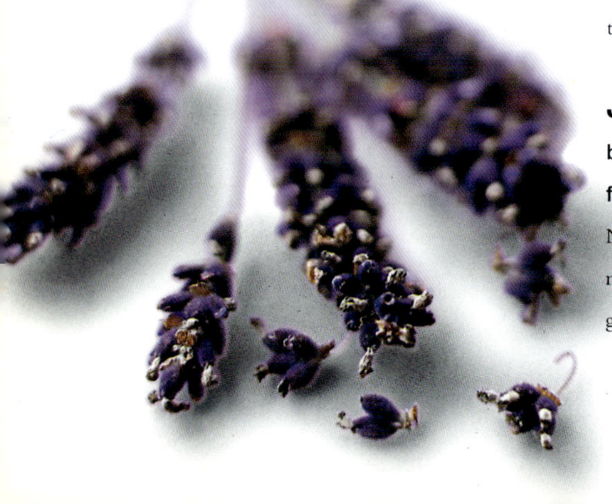

Geranium

botanical name *Pelargonium graveolens*

family *Geraniaceae*

With its serrated, heart-shaped leaves and brightly coloured flowers, geranium is a popular household plant. The light green essential oil comes from the aromatic leaves, and has a rose-like aroma. It is often used to dilute the very expensive rose oil in perfumes and other beauty products.

properties analgesic, antibacterial, antidepressant, antifungal, anti-inflammatory, antispasmodic, antiseptic, astringent, decongestant, deodorant, digestive stimulant, insect repellent, relaxant

uses *body* use in instances of inflammation, acne, herpes, diarrhoea, varicose veins, urinary tract infections and menstrual problems *mind* alleviates grief, anger, moodiness, depression, anxiety *spirit* brings order and balance, restores harmony

cautions avoid the essential oil during the first three months of pregnancy

Jasmine

botanical name *Jasminum grandiflorum*

family *Oleaceae*

Native to China and India, this creeping vine is a member of the olive family. The plant has dark-green leaves and intoxicatingly fragrant white flowers from which is extracted the essential oil. Jasmine is one of the most expensive perfume ingredients. The flowers are used to scent China tea, and garlands of them are used in the Buddhist religion to symbolize respect.

properties pain reliever, antidepressant, antiseptic, antispasmodic, anti-inflammatory, expectorant, uterine tonic, aphrodisiac

uses *body* beneficial in skincare, particularly of dry and sensitive skin, it also increases skin elasticity, eases period pains and muscular aches and pains *mind* helps relieve apathy, indifference, listlessness, post-natal depression, stress-related disorders *spirit* liberates imagination, provokes fantasies, releases and encourages inner desires

cautions avoid the essential oil when pregnant

Lavender

botanical name *Lavandula angustifolia*

family *Lamiaceae*

This herb is extensively cultivated in England and France. It has grey-green leaves and fragrant blue-violet flowers borne on long spikes. The flowers and stems are used dried and fresh in cooking and in infusions. The essential oil is obtained from the plant's flowering tops. Lavender has been a popular fragrance for centuries and is used in

a variety of beauty and household products.
properties analgesic, antimicrobial, antiseptic, anti-inflammatory, antispasmodic, calming and sedative, decongestant, tonic, immunity booster
uses *body* skin rejuvenator, normalizes dry and oily skin, helps psoriasis and eczema, eases high blood pressure, asthma, arthritis and rheumatism *mind* eases tension headaches, agitation and anxiety and insomnia, is useful in treatment of depression, fear, grief, indecision and emotional conflict, and extreme mood swings *spirit* restores peace and tranquillity, eases the trauma of change, helps the individual become receptive to new ideas and experiences
cautions avoid using the essential oil during the first three months of pregnancy

Neroli

botanical name *Citrus aurantium*
family *Rutaceae*

The essential oil neroli is distilled from the blossoms of the bitter orange tree, an evergreen citrus tree native to Asia but nowadays cultivated extensively in the Mediterranean region. The expressed oil is produced in Israel, Cyprus, Brazil and the US. Neroli has a soft, floral fragrance, and is the most costly of the various orange oils.
properties antidepressant, antiseptic, deodorant, digestive, sedative, tonic, aphrodisiac
uses *body* beneficial in skincare, improves elasticity, is regenerative, aids in the healing of scars, thread veins and the stretch marks of pregnancy *mind* relieves hysteria, anxiety, depression, insomnia *spirit* calms, aids confidence
cautions no known contraindications for the essential oil

Rose

botanical name *Rosa damascena*
family *Rosaceae*

In the Valley of the Roses in Bulgaria, the highly prized damask rose is cultivated. The plant is picked at sunrise to maximize its oil yield, known as rose otto or attar of roses. The oil is distilled from the intoxicatingly fragrant petals. Other varieties of rose are also appreciated for their fragrance, either as fresh or dried flowers, or as slightly cheaper essential oils.
properties antidepressant, antibacterial, astringent, anti-infectious, anti-inflammatory, cleansing, sexual tonic, aphrodisiac
uses *body* balances hormones, regulates menstruation, is helpful in cases of frigidity or impotence, improves the circulation, regulates the heart, rejuvenates and regenerates the skin *mind* eases guilt, jealousy, grief, resentment, depression, insomnia, tension headaches *spirit* heals the heart and emotions, re-establishes connections with loved ones, brings a sense of deep relaxation and inner peace
cautions avoid the essential oil during the first three months of pregnancy

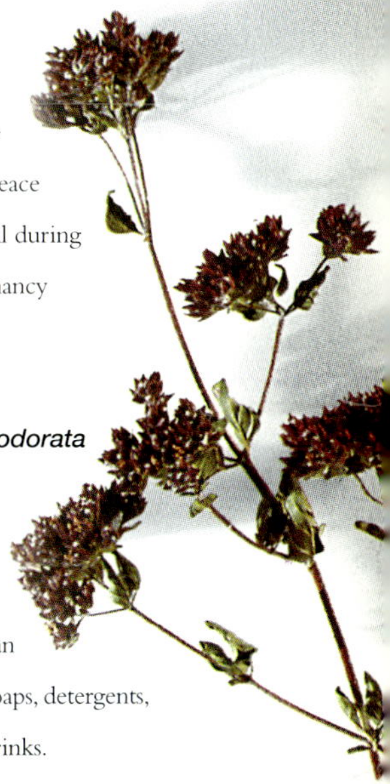

Ylang ylang

botanical name *Cananga odorata*
family *Annonaceae*

This glossy-leaved evergreen tree is native to tropical Asia. The thick yellow petals yield an exotic oil used in cosmetics, soaps, detergents, lotions, perfumes, foods and drinks.
properties antidepressant, antiseptic, antispasmodic, calming and sedative, aphrodisiac, circulatory stimulant, reproductive tonic
uses *body* regulates cardiac and respiratory rhythm, relaxes muscles, is a useful tonic for dry hair and scalp, stimulates hair growth, and soothes dry, inflamed skin *mind* helpful in cases of irritability, fear, introversion, shyness, stress-related disorders *spirit* opens the heart, making deeper understanding possible, creates feelings of peace and warmth
cautions use the essential oil in moderation, excessive use of ylang ylang can lead to nausea and headaches

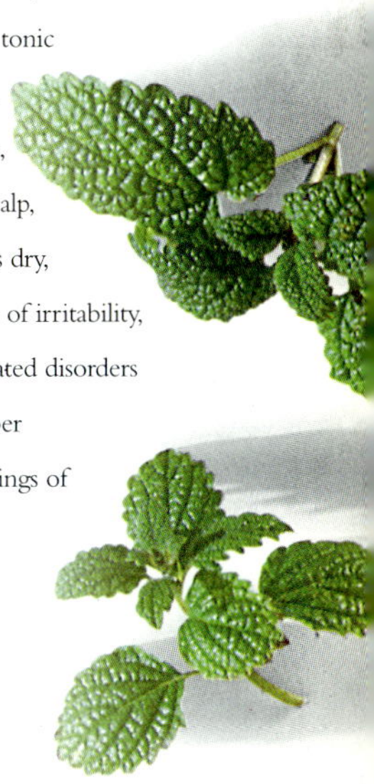

scents from the herb garden

Basil

botanical name *Ocimum basilicum*

family *Lamiaceae*

The leaves of this popular culinary herb are used for their sweet, refreshing aroma and flavour. Basil essential oil is distilled from the whole plant.

properties analgesic, antibacterial, antifungal, anti-inflammatory, antiseptic, antispasmodic, antiviral, digestive tonic, expectorant, nervous system regulator, purifier, stimulant

uses *body* eases indigestion, sinus congestion, arthritis, tired muscles *mind* alleviates anxiety, fear, jealousy, indecision, confusion, exhaustion *spirit* enhances inspiration and gives spiritual protection

cautions always use the essential oil following the recommended dosage, do not use the oil during pregnancy

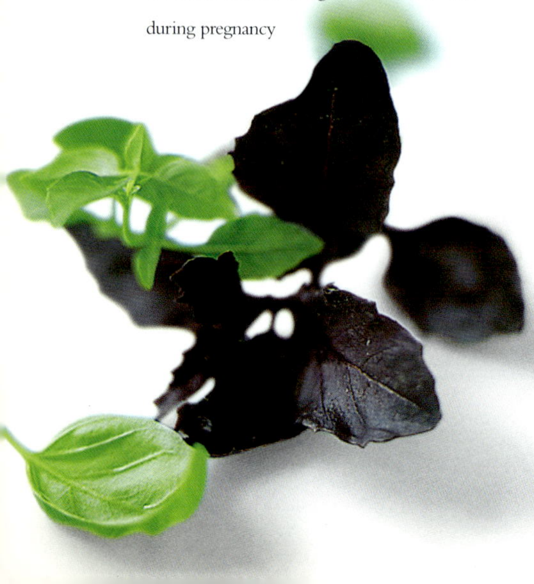

Clary sage

botanical name *Salvia sclarea*

family *Lamiaceae*

This hardy herb is found in most parts of the world. It has broad, wrinkled leaves and long stalks that bear small blue, pink or white flowers. The essential oil is distilled from the dried plant and is used in eau de Cologne and lavender water as well as muscatel wines and vermouth.

properties antifungal, anti-infectious, detoxicant, antispasmodic, decongestant, regenerative, euphoric, aphrodisiac, relaxant, sedative, tonic

uses *body* helpful for females with reproductive problems, relaxes spasms in asthma *mind* relieves extreme fear, panic, post-natal depression *spirit* encourages vivid dreams and dream recall

cautions prolonged inhalation of the essential oil may cause drowsiness, avoid during pregnancy, avoid alcohol consumption before and after use

Coriander

botanical name *Coriandrum sativum*

family *Umbelliferae*

Native to Europe and Asia, this herb has bright green, delicate leaves, with dainty whitish-pink flowers. The fresh leaves (known by their Spanish name, cilantro, in the United States) are used in cooking and in medicinal infusions. The small seeds are dried and used in cooking, crushed to form spice, or distilled to produce the essential oil.

properties antispasmodic, antirheumatic, digestive, euphoric, stimulant, tonic, warming

uses *body* eases arthritis, sprains, strains, muscle spasms *mind* relieves worry, anxiety, depression *spirit* encourages inner peace and creativity

cautions the essential oil is a possible skin irritant, use only in recommended amounts, can also be stupefying in large doses

Fennel

botanical name *Foeniculum vulgare*

family *Umbelliferae*

This perennial herb from the Mediterranean has dark-green feathery leaves and clusters of small yellow flowers. The essential oil, which is distilled from the seeds, has a sweet aniseed-like aroma.

properties analgesic, antibacterial, antifungal, anti-inflammatory, decongestant, digestive, laxative

uses *body* promotes milk flow, eases menstrual pains, menopause symptoms and ovary problems *mind* relieves insecurity and pessimism *spirit* inspires courage and creative self-expression

cautions use only in recommended dosages, avoid if suffering from epilepsy or if pregnant

Marjoram

botanical name *Origanum marjorana*

family *Lamiaceae*

Sweet marjoram is a popular culinary herb and has a reputation for promoting longevity. The plant grows mainly in the Mediterranean regions and has tiny white or pink flowers: the oil is distilled from the plant's leaves and flowers.

properties analgesic, antibacterial, anti-infectious, antispasmodic, digestive stimulant, expectorant, diuretic, tonic, calming, strongly sedative, warming

uses *body* relieves coughs, cold sores, intestinal spasms, heartburn, colic, muscle spasms and sprains *mind* eases grief, anger, moodiness, insomnia *spirit* promotes a sense of calm and inner strength

cautions avoid the essential oil during pregnancy and if asthmatic, do not use for depression

Melissa

botanical name *Melissa officinalis*

family *Lamiaceae*

Also known as lemon balm, melissa is a small herb with tiny white flowers that originates from southern Europe. A daily drink of tea prepared from the fresh leaves is supposed to encourage longevity. When the leaves are distilled they produce a pale oil with a crisp, lemony scent.

properties antidepressant, anti-inflammatory, antispasmodic, antiviral, calming and sedative

uses *body* relieves painful periods, vomiting, nervous indigestion *mind* eases grief, tension headaches, insomnia, hysteria, panic, anxiety *spirit* brings understanding and awareness

cautions do not expose the skin to sunlight or a sunbed for two hours after using the essential oil, pure melissa oil is difficult to obtain and some cheaper brands contain skin irritants

Peppermint

botanical name *Mentha piperita*

family *Lamiaceae*

This small herb has dark-green leaves with serrated edges and small purplish flowers from which its essential oil is distilled. Peppermint's medicinal qualities have long been appreciated, and the essential oil is a handy first aid standby.

properties analgesic, antibacterial, antifungal, anti-inflammatory, antimigraine, antispasmodic, insect repellent, reproductive stimulant

uses *body* eases indigestion, nausea, travel sickness, diarrhoea, clears congestion, relieves bronchitis, asthma, sinusitis and colds *mind* alleviates anger, guilt, apathy, mental fatigue, depression, inability to concentrate, shock *spirit* revitalizes the inner-self, increases ability to digest new experiences

cautions use the essential oil sparingly; keep to recommended dilution, avoid during pregnancy, a strong mental stimulant – avoid at bedtime

Rosemary

botanical name *Rosmarinus officinalis*

family *Lamiaceae*

Native to the Mediterranean regions, this aromatic evergreen shrub has needle-shaped leaves and pale blue flowers. It has a rich history of both culinary and medicinal use. The essential oil is obtained from the flowers and leaves.

properties analgesic, antibacterial, antifungal, anti-infectious, anti-inflammatory, antispasmodic, antiviral, astringent, cleansing, detoxicant, digestive, diuretic, sexual tonic, stimulant, warming

uses *body* useful in the treatment of respiratory problems, rheumatic and muscular pain, arthritis, congestive headaches, constipation, indigestion and poor circulation *mind* eases depression, and mental exhaustion through overwork, improves memory *spirit* opens the heart, increases sensitivity, creativity and awareness of inner potential

cautions avoid using the essential oil during pregnancy or if suffering from epilepsy or from high blood pressure, a strong mental stimulant – avoid at bedtime

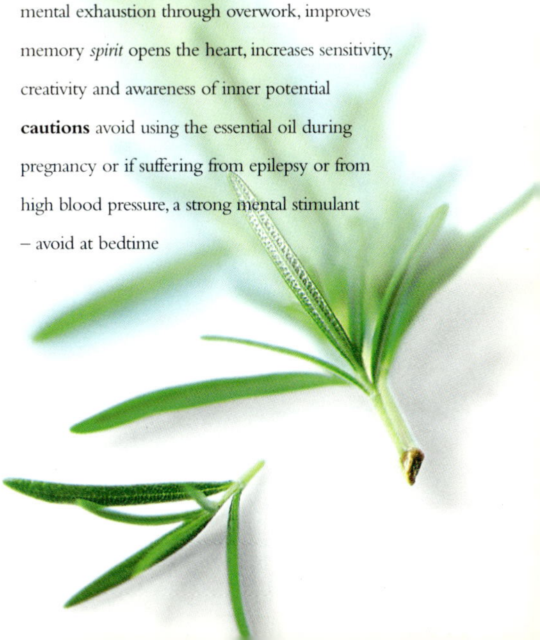

zesty and refreshing scents

Bergamot

botanical name *Citrus bergamia*

family *Rutaceae*

The essential oil of this ornamental citrus tree is expressed from the peel of the inedible fruit. The oil is used in eau de Cologne, and the leaves are used to flavour Earl Grey tea.

properties antibacterial, anti-infectious, antiseptic, antispasmodic, antiviral, calming

uses *body* eases digestive problems, useful in treating oily skin *mind* combats grief, anxiety, depression *spirit* increases self-confidence

cautions do not expose the skin to sunlight for two hours after using the essential oil

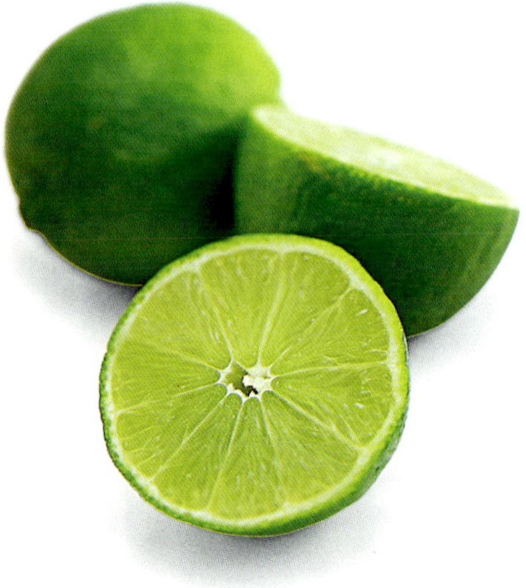

Grapefruit

botanical name *Citrus paradis*

family *Rutaceae*

The delicious, large, yellow fruits of this tropical tree are eaten whole or used for their juice. The yellow essential oil is obtained from the peel and is used in perfumery.

properties antidepressant, antiseptic, diuretic, digestive, stimulant, tonic

uses *body* effective in treatment of oily skin, cellulite, obesity *mind* alleviates depression, melancholy *spirit* uplifts and revives

cautions use the essential oil within six months, seek medical advice before using if taking immuno-suppressant drugs

Cypress

botanical name *Cupressus sempervirens*

family *Cupressaceae*

Some of these tall, evergreen conifers are believed to be more than 3000 years old. The essential oil is distilled from the tree's leaves, cones and twigs while the durable wood is used in furniture making and ship building.

properties antibacterial, anti-infectious, antispasmodic, astringent, calming, deodorant

uses *body* aids respiratory disorders, asthma, tickly coughs, improves greasy hair and skin, acne, acts as hormone regulator for menstrual problems *mind* eases grief, insomnia, mental sluggishness *spirit* soothes in stressful times of transition, particularly during difficult change such as a divorce or bereavement

cautions avoid using the essential oil during pregnancy

Juniper

botanical name *Juniperus communis*

family *Cupressaceae*

The juniper tree is a small evergreen from the same family as cypress. It has short spiny leaves and blue-black berries from which is distilled the sweetly fragrant essential oil. Juniper berries are also used to make gin.

properties analgesic, antiseptic, detoxifying, digestive tonic, diuretic, purifying, stimulant

uses *body* aids acne and oily skin problems, cystitis, water retention, cellulite *mind* eases guilt, jealousy, emotional exhaustion, insomnia *spirit* helps to reconnect with inner vision

cautions avoid the essential oil during pregnancy, do not use with conditions associated with kidney disease

Lemon

botanical name *Citrus limon*

family *Rutaceae*

The lemon tree is native to Asia but grows wild in many Mediterranean countries, and is also cultivated in many parts of the world, including the Americas. Lemons are rich in vitamin C and their juice and peel are widely used in cooking. The essential oil is expressed from the fruit's peel.

properties anti-anaemic, antibacterial, anti-infectious, anti-inflammatory, antiseptic

uses *body* relieves coughs, colds, respiratory infections, combats greasy skin and hair, acts as a detoxicant *mind* alleviates sluggishness and indecision, eases depression, apathy and fear *spirit* brings freshness, clarity

cautions do not expose the skin to sunlight or a sunbed for two hours after using the essential oil, like all citrus oils, the oil has a short shelf life: use within six months

Lime

botanical name *Citrus aurantifolia*

family *Rutaceae*

The smallest member of the true citrus family, the lime resembles the lemon, but its fruits are rounder and greener. Today it is extensively grown in Italy and tropical America. In the 19th century English sailors were made to eat limes to prevent scurvy, thus earning the tag "limeys". The oil is expressed from the fruit's peel.

properties antiseptic, astringent, restorative

uses *body* relieves pain from insect bites, acts as a detoxicant and appetite stimulant, reduces greasy skin and scalp *mind* relieves listlessness, depression *spirit* uplifts the spirits

cautions do not expose the skin to sunlight or a sunbed for two hours after using the essential oil, use the oil within six months

Orange

botanical name *Citrus sinensis*

family *Rutaceae*

Native to China, oranges were probably known to the Ancient Greeks and may have been the mythical Golden Apples of the Hesperides, and today the evergreen tree is cultivated in many parts of the world. Oranges have a long tradition in both therapeutic and culinary use. The golden yellow essential oil is obtained from the peel.

properties antidepressant, antispasmodic, antiseptic, sedative, tonic, mellow, warming

uses *body* improves poor circulation, eases indigestion, colds and flu *mind* helps alleviate depression, sadness, nervous tension, stress-related disorders *spirit* restores optimism, enthusiasm and joy, encourages spontaneity

cautions as with other citrus oils, do not expose the skin to sunlight or a sunbed for two hours after using the essential oil, may cause dermatitis

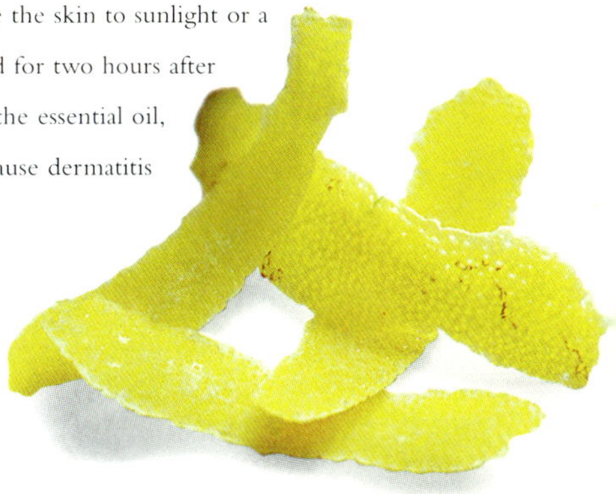

Pine

botanical name *Pinus sylvestris*

family *Pinaceae*

The pine tree grows widely throughout northern Europe and Russia. This tall tree has a reddish, fissured bark and long stiff needle-like leaves with brown cones. The essential oil comes from the leaves, while the dried bark and cones can be used in potpourri.

properties analgesic, antibacterial, antifungal, strongly antiseptic, deodorant, cleansing

uses *body* fights respiratory tract infections, hay fever, cystitis, rheumatism *mind* eases melancholy, pessimism, fatigue *spirit* inspires and revitalizes, cleanses and opens up the aura

cautions no known contraindications

exotic aromas

Black pepper

botanical name *Piper nigrum*

family *Piperaceae*

Cultivated in India and Malaysia, the ripe red berries of this climbing vine are picked and dried, turning them black. Peppercorns are used both whole and ground or distilled to produce the essential oil.

properties analgesic, antidepressant, expectorant

uses *body* relieves coughs, colds, poor circulation *mind* eases suppressed anger, relieves indifference *spirit* brings courage, renews enthusiasm

cautions can cause skin irritation

Cinnamon

botanical name *Cinnamomum zeylanicum*

family *Lauraceae*

The inner bark of this tropical tree is dried to produce quills of cinnamon spice. Both the leaves and the bark produce an essential oil.

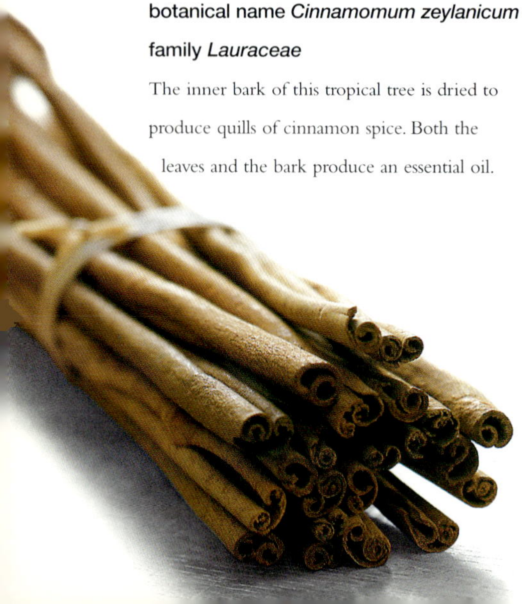

properties antifungal, antimicrobial, antiseptic, antispasmodic, circulatory stimulant, digestive

uses *body* revives sluggish digestive, lymphatic and/or circulatory system, helps fight infections of the skin *mind* relieves mental fatigue and aids concentration *spirit* awakens the body and mind

cautions the bark oil cannot be used on the skin, the leaf oil can be, but in concentrations of 0.5 per cent or less, avoid during pregnancy

Cloves

botanical name *Syzygium aromaticum*

family *Myrtaceae*

Native to the Molucca Islands, the brilliant red flower buds of this slender, evergreen tree turn red-brown when dried.The essential oil is distilled from the buds, leaves and stalks, and the dried buds are used in infusions and cooking.

properties analgesic, antibiotic, anaesthetic, antispasmodic, antioxidant, antiseptic, antiviral

uses *body* useful as preventative treatment for colds and flu, clears blocked sinuses *mind* eases mental fatigue and mental restlessness, assists concentration *spirit* promotes sense of wellbeing

cautions can irritate the skin and mucous membranes, use the oil in low concentrations, as a vaporizer, avoid use during pregnancy

Eucalyptus

botanical name *Eucalyptus globulus*

family *Myrtaceae*

Native to Australia, the leaves of these trees have traditionally been smoked to alleviate asthma, and bound onto wounds to help them heal. The essential oil is distilled from the leaves.

properties analgesic, anti-infectious, antiseptic, decongestant, digestive stimulant

uses *body* fevers, infectious illness, respiratory conditions, coughs, colds *mind* extreme mood swings, mental exhaustion, poor concentration *spirit* creates a feeling of freedom and space

cautions do not use with young children, or if suffering from high blood pressure or epilepsy, do not use in higher concentrations than 1 per cent, may counteract homeopathic remedies

Frankincense

botanical name *Boswellia carteri*

family *Burseraceae*

These pink-flowering trees grow in north-east Africa and Arabia. The tree exudes a white serum, which solidifies on exposure to the air. These solid "tears" are distilled for their oil.

properties analgesic, antiseptic, anticatarrhal, antidepressant, anti-inflammatory, energizing

uses *body* relieves asthma and respiratory tract disorders, rejuvenates aging skin *mind* eases anger, anxiety, nervous tension *spirit* awakens the soul to higher levels of consciousness
cautions no known contraindications

Ginger

botanical name *Zingiber officinale*
family *Zingiberaceae*

Native to Asia, the essential oil is distilled from the creeping rhizome of this herb, which is also used both fresh and dried in the kitchen.
properties analgesic, anticatarrhal, digestive stimulant, expectorant, general and sexual tonic
uses *body* reduces flatulence, constipation, warms stiff joints *mind* combats self-doubt, emotional coldness *spirit* builds self-confidence
cautions possible skin irritant, should not be used in higher concentration than 1 per cent

Myrrh

botanical name *Commiphora myrrha*
family *Burseraceae*

This small tree grows in the deserts of Africa and Arabia. The wood secretes a resin that hardens into small "tears" on exposure to the air, from which is produced the essential oil.
properties anti-inflammatory, antiseptic, astringent, cooling, expectorant, sedative, tonic
uses *body* promotes healthy teeth and gums, eases throat and mouth inflammations, aids in skincare *mind* helps in states of heated emotion *spirit* soothes and calms, expands awareness
cautions avoid during pregnancy

Nutmeg

botanical name *Myristica fragrans*
family *Myristicaceae*

Grown in Indonesia, Sri Lanka and the West Indies, the ripe fruits split open to reveal the kernel (nutmeg) wrapped in its net-like arils (mace). The nutmeg and mace are used dried in cooking. The oil comes from crushed nutmeg.
properties analgesic, antiseptic, antispasmodic, digestive, stimulant, tonic, warming
uses *body* revives sluggish digestion, eases nausea, vomiting, bad breath *mind* relieves tension, sexual inhibitions *spirit* aids intimacy with loved ones
cautions avoid during pregnanc, always use in concentrations of 0.5 per cent or less, over-use can cause nausea, hallucinations and stupor

Sandalwood

botanical name *Santalum album*
family *Santalaceae*

This slow-growing evergreen tree is native to India, where it is a protected species. When the mature trees are cut down, termites are used to remove the sapwood, leaving the fragrant heartwood, which produces the essential oil.
properties anti-infectious, diuretic, immune stimulant, moisturizing, sedative
uses *body* combats urinary infections (such as cystitis), acts as a digestive aid, relieves nausea *mind* alleviates fear, guilt, insomnia and stress *spirit* uplifts and revives, aids dreaming
cautions inhalation may cause drowsiness, avoid alcohol consumption before or after use

Tea tree

botanical name *Melaleuca alternifolia*
family *Myrtaceae*

This small yellow-flowered tree is native to Australia, and was long used by the Australian Aborigines for its many medicinal properties.
properties analgesic, antibacterial, antiseptic, antiviral, expectorant, immune stimulant
uses *body* helps in the treatment of respiratory disorders, Candida albicans (thrush), infected wounds *mind* eases shock, nervous exhaustion *spirit* strengthens and protects, deeply cleansing
cautions no known contraindications

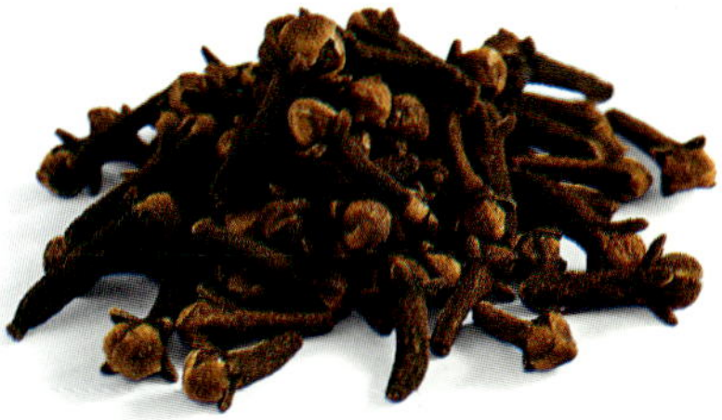

index

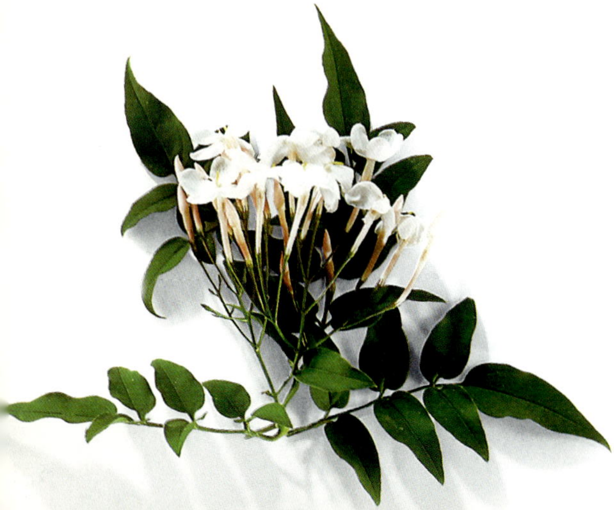

Picture credits:
Sue Atkinson p57; Simon Bottomley p14, 16, 23r, 29l & br, 53; Martin Brigdale p1, 56, 58, 59, 61; Nik Cole p49; Nikki Dowey p40, 46; Gus Filgate p54; Michelle Garrett p2, 10, 12, 15b, 17tr, 19br, tl & tr, 21, 23l, 24, 25, 26, 29tr, 30tl & r, 31, 34, 36tl, 37, 38, 39br, 43tl, tr & bl, 44, 45l, 47, 50, 51, 52, 54; Alistair Hughes p8, 39tr; Andrea Jones p27, 36bl; Don Last p6, 22; William Lingwood p43br, 60, 63; Debbie Patterson p7, 8, 9, 19bl; Spike Powell p48; and Polly Wreford p4, 6, 11, 13, 15t, 20, 33.